W9-BRB-802

Praise for

The Jerusalem Diet

"Practical and simple, the Jerusalem Diet is a great prescription for my patients who need to lose weight. With the Jerusalem Diet they can keep the weight off for life. I am excited to be able to give this to my patients."

—KENT G. ROBERSON, MD, Family Health Center

"Ted Haggard has effectively lent his gift of making the complicated easy to the quagmire of diet and exercise. Not only is this book practical, it is actually fun. There is no longer any reason to hold back on your health, because this approach is healthy, effective, and completely painless!"

—LISA BEVERE, author, *Kissed the Girls and Made Them Cry, Out of Control and Loving It!* and *Be Angry But Don't Blow It*

"During my fifteen years of practicing medicine, I have counseled many people in nutrition and weight loss. I have been gravely disappointed in what medical and nutritional science have had to offer. I have seen diets and medicine work for a while but usually without sustained results. *The Jerusalem Diet* offers new hope with a practical strategy that allows people to never be more than one pound away from their goal weight. It gives great hope in weight loss and maintaining what has been lost. Thank you, Ted Haggard, for bringing freedom to an area that has caused so much bondage! This is truly a framework for success."

—THOMAS A. HENDERSON, MD, Advantage Inpatient Medical
   Specialists

"This book is not another fad diet plan but a lifestyle approach that will help put you on the road to good health."

—CHRISTOPHER R. COLE, MD, F.A.C.C., Director, Colorado
   Cardiac Alliance Research Institute

The
Jerusalem
Diet

ALSO BY TED HAGGARD

Foolish No More

Dog Training, Fly Fishing, and Sharing Christ in the Twenty-First Century

Letters from Home

The Life-Giving Church

Simple Prayers for a Powerful Life

Primary Purpose

Taking It to the Streets

Loving Your City into the Kingdom (with Jack Hayford)

Confident Parents, Exceptional Teens (with John Bolin)

The
Jerusalem
Diet

The "ONE DAY" APPROACH to Reach Your Ideal Weight—and STAY THERE

TED HAGGARD

Foreword by Larry Gee, M.D.

WATERBROOK
PRESS

THE JERUSALEM DIET
PUBLISHED BY WATERBROOK PRESS
12265 Oracle Boulevard, Suite 200
Colorado Springs, Colorado 80921
A division of Random House, Inc.

ISBN 1-4000-7220-4

Library of Congress Cataloging-in-Publication Data
Haggard, Ted.
    The Jerusalem diet : the "one day" approach to reach your ideal weight—and stay there / Ted Haggard.—1st ed.
        p. cm.
    Includes bibliographical references and index.
    ISBN 1-4000-7220-4
    1. Reducing diets. I. Title.
RM222.2.H218 2005
613.2'5—dc22

                                    2005025667

Printed in the United States of America
2005—First Edition

10 9 8 7 6 5 4 3 2 1

＊

⟨∽⟩⟨∽⟩

This book is dedicated to my wife, Gayle, who has insisted that fruits and vegetables reign on our family's table, that whole-wheat bread replace white bread, that water and juices prevail against soft drinks, and that balanced "real food" meals carry the day over junk food. Throughout our marriage, books about nutrition, diet, exercise, and disease prevention have rested on our nightstands and coffee tables. Gayle is incredible! She weighs less and looks better today, after giving birth to five children, than she did when we married twenty-seven years ago. Because of Gayle, our family is healthy and strong. Because of Gayle, the Jerusalem Diet is a natural as a health-weight plan for me. We all thank you, Gayle.

Contents

Foreword

by Larry Gee, MD

I am a family-practice doctor with a strong interest in health promotion and preventive medicine. I have had the privilege of working and teaching about health all over the world.

When I first heard that Pastor Ted Haggard was teaching about dieting, to be honest, I was a bit skeptical. He has been my pastor since 1996, and I had the privilege of watching him up close when we traveled together on a mission trip to Nepal. I enjoy his teaching on many topics, and he always has appeared healthy—so he must be doing something right. But what does a pastor know about nutrition and dieting?

Unfortunately, the same question could be asked of many doctors! As a whole, physicians tend to be some of the more unhealthy people I know. We do a lot of health and diet education but may not practice it ourselves.

When Pastor Ted asked me to review *The Jerusalem Diet,* I thought it would be a great chance to ensure he didn't make a fool of himself by writing on a topic he doesn't know much about. As I dived into the book, however, I was surprised to find out how simple and practical the plan was. I told him later, "This is so simple even a doctor can follow it!"

I especially appreciated the chapter called "I Love Food!" So much of life is centered around food, as I was reminded again at a recent family reunion. Every decade, Americans are eating more, exercising less, and getting fatter and fatter. Many Americans carry thirty to a hundred pounds of extra weight. Because of this, they suffer from a host of obesity-related diseases and disabilities, and they cannot function as well as they would like. They cannot keep up with their kids and do all the things God has called them to do.

Every time I return to the United States after being out of the country, I am overwhelmed by our obesity. Sadly, the Chinese and other people in many parts of the world are catching up with us as the American fast-food diet and sedentary lifestyle spread.

My ideal weight is 195 pounds. Since high school, I had ballooned to a high of 235 pounds. I had worked my way back to 215 pounds but was having a really hard time getting below this. (My kids tell me I am in pretty good shape for a fat guy.) I am a lot like Pastor Ted in that I don't like to follow strict diet plans and don't have time to count calories or find special foods. I, too, am a busy father. How would I ever have time to go to diet group meetings? Like Ted and many others, I am also not very disciplined. I can make myself work out, but I have a very hard time controlling food intake.

As I read the manuscript, I realized the Jerusalem Diet was something I could follow. I decided to give it a try to see if I could get down to my ideal weight once again. In just seven weeks I have been surprised at how effective and easy it is. I have consistently lost one pound per week, and I feel better already. I am excited that I have almost achieved my New Year's resolution to be under 205 in 2005.

I love how flexible this plan is. When I went to my family reunion, I decided to enjoy the time and not follow the diet. I didn't weigh myself at all. I thought when I got back I would really pay the price. But I had to do only one Fat Day—eating fruits, vegetables, nuts, and seeds, drinking only water, and exercising at least one hour—and I was back on track. At two recent birthday dinners I ate whatever I wanted and again just had to do one Fat Day.

I actually enjoy Fat Days, because I still eat a lot of good food. As you read the book and start the diet, you will be surprised how well you feel eating good food. In time, your taste buds will desire more and more healthy food. I am reminded of the cartoon showing a doctor telling a patient what he should eat. The patient responds, "That is not food. That is what food eats!"

I also appreciate Ted's exhortation to exercise. The bottom line with weight loss is you must burn up more calories than you take in. There are all sorts of advertised shortcuts for this, but they never work without complications. As you move your life toward more regular exercise, you will start feeling better and be able to do more, even if you are still over your ideal weight. The best exercise is the one you like doing. I personally prefer mountain biking, because it is a lot like the Jerusalem Diet—you only have to work hard and discipline yourself for a short time, and then you have a fun downhill roller-coaster ride.

By the way, a good exercise program consists of ten minutes of stretching, thirty minutes of aerobic exercise, and twenty minutes of weightlifting. You need to include all three to be in really good shape. Studies show that morning exercise programs are more likely to be continued than afternoon or evening ones, because when you get home from work, it is too easy not to work out. I also encourage you to find physical activities that include your whole family.

As a physician, I think there are very few people who could not safely follow the Jerusalem Diet. If you have special health problems, such as heart disease, hypertension, or diabetes, you should consult your doctor and continue to follow his or her diet recommendations as you integrate this lifestyle change. As Pastor Ted says, this is not so much a diet as it is a way to live healthier and practice some of the things you probably already know you should be doing.

You also can apply many of these principles to help your kids keep their ideal weight, but be careful about overfocusing on their weight, since it is ever changing as they grow taller.

We have a choice as we go through life. We can maintain physical, emotional, and spiritual fitness so we can function to our fullest into our seventies and eighties, or we can have more and more disabilities, do less and less, and die in our fifties or sixties. God wants us to enjoy life and to stay healthy.

As you lose those extra pounds, you will experience life to the fullest. This book, if you follow it, will help you achieve and maintain your goal.

I am glad you picked up this book, and I hope you will join me on the journey toward ideal weight and healthy living.

Hot Fudge Sundaes Are Good for You!

People have been asking me to write this diet book for years.

I do a lot of traveling and speaking, and since 1998 I've occasionally discussed the health plan that is now called the Jerusalem Diet. (I'll tell the whole story behind my discovery of the diet in chapters 2 and 3.)

"You *have* to turn this into a book," people would say. So here we go.

At its core the Jerusalem Diet is not just about eating but about a lifestyle that's easily communicated and understood. It's a way of doing and being—a world-view, a mentality about food and health.

All the famous diets you are aware of can work with this idea. The Jerusalem Diet is simply a framework, and a flexible one at that. It offers a plan, but you can adjust it to develop your own system for eating, exercising, and enjoying your life.

You should know that I'm not a physician—I'm a pastor. While the information in this book has been researched and tested by personal experience, what I have to tell you does not have the authority of an MD. If you need a doctor, talk to a doctor. But as a pastor, I often work as a life coach. It is my responsibility to figure out general trends in people's lives and help them live better, longer, healthier. Often that means talking about their families, jobs, and spirituality, but it also means talking about things like food and exercise.

I have personal reasons for being interested in this subject as well: both my mother and father were obese and died early because of it. Several other members of my family struggle with weight issues, and in the fall of 1998 I began to struggle with extra pounds of my own. It frightened me—I want to live my full life span, and I want to feel good.

Also—and if you haven't been around the Christian culture much, this may strike you as strange—pastors are the single fattest group of people I know! Food is such a big part of church life—potluck dinners, pizza parties, Sunday suppers, and those famous holiday banquets with piles and piles of food. We love to eat, and I love that we love to eat. But for some of us, all this food becomes a problem.

The Jerusalem Diet changed my life and helped establish the culture of health that is in New Life Church, where I pastor in Colorado Springs. We don't talk about it much, but the people who are in leadership model it. They are not "beautiful" people who are overly conscious of their appearance; they are just ordinary people who look healthy.

I had been using the Jerusalem Diet for several years but had never thought of teaching it until one evening when I was the after-dinner speaker at a banquet for the pastors of one of the largest church denominations in America. I was seated with the president, and as a courtesy, I asked him if there was anything specific he wanted me to say in my speech.

"Thanks, Ted," he said. "Actually, I invited you because I do want you to talk about something."

"What do you have in mind?" I wondered why he hadn't mentioned the topic to me earlier.

"Ted, this will be easy for you. Just speak from your heart and experience."

"So, what do you want me to talk about?"

"Look around," he responded.

I didn't see anything but a banquet room and pastors from all over America eating with their spouses and friends.

"Look again."

I did, and this time I saw it. *Everyone* in the room was overweight. I turned to him in horror. "You can't ask me to address this subject at your national banquet!"

"This is the acceptable sin in our movement," he said. "Our leaders are so fat that they're sick and dying early. Our churches are a disgrace, because everyone on the platform on Sundays is fat."

I laughed and said, "I do have a plan that makes fat people happy. And when they are happy and hopeful, they can lose weight and improve their lives."

"I know. That's why you are here," he answered, smiling.

That occasion was the first time I taught the Jerusalem Diet in public. I did it on the condition that I could speak to the same group the next year. I taught the simplicity of the program you are going to read about. Then I left for twelve months.

At the next year's banquet, I couldn't believe my eyes. There were a few heavy people in the room, but not nearly as many. The group seemed happier, laughing and enjoying their meal. They looked better and appeared to feel better too. Interestingly, many of them came up to me and told me about sicknesses they had been struggling with the year before that were now gone. For many, the Jerusalem Diet had given them the hope they needed for a new start.

Yes, the Jerusalem Diet works, but it is not a quick fix. If you want an instant, easy reversal of the damage you've done to your body over many years, this plan may not be right for you. The Jerusalem Diet—although easy—requires patience. It takes time for your diet to change, your weight to reduce gradually, your body shape to adjust to your ideal weight, your muscles to tone, and your metabolism to increase so that food doesn't always make you fat. It requires that you be loving and patient with yourself as you become your best.

I think you will love this plan!

I've presented this concept to groups of leaders and other busy people. In every case it has given them a way to address their weight concerns without radically unbalancing their world.

The challenge with any diet is sticking to it. All diet plans work. If you hear about a new diet, buy the book and start the program. That diet will work for you until you don't want to do it anymore. Then you'll quit or start another diet, and the new diet will work too—until you get bored and give up. We've all done this. For people who stay on Atkins, Atkins works. People who stick with Weight Watchers have success. But very few people can stay on the same plan successfully year after year.

The problem—the wonderful, wonderful problem!—is that we have so much variety in food and one opportunity after another to eat. We can eat almost anything we want. If we are hungry for a doughnut, it's no problem to go to Krispy Kreme and eat three or four or eight doughnuts in one sitting. If we feel like having a burger and fries, four bucks will get us a quick, tasty slab of meat grilled to perfection and served in a toasted bun—with mustard and ketchup oozing out the sides.

What I will do is give you a plan that allows you to enjoy the variety of food that's available and also refines your approach to that food. I want you to enjoy the food you like without guilt. I also want you to avoid favorite foods for short periods when you need to. I will give you a plan that doesn't embarrass you or force you to embarrass others. A plan that inspires hope instead of dread, that fosters success instead of failure, that challenges in a productive way and is actually pleasant.

Being overweight is the most obvious dilemma, but being underweight is a problem too. Most of the examples in this book deal with people who need to lose weight. But these ideas also work for people who are too thin.

In short, I want to improve your life!

So here's the deal: I am going to give you a diet with specific nutrition and exercise guidelines. You can follow it easily. But mostly, this overarching, big umbrella idea will assist you for the rest of your life. It's easy, and it works.

In this book you'll learn how to

- slowly incorporate a fitness mentality that is easy to follow, as you…
- relax and enjoy the food you like without nagging guilt, while you…
- pragmatically address your health concerns, whether you're overweight or underweight, and…
- shift the trajectory of your life toward total well-being.

New world-views need time to percolate. If you are going to incorporate a big, new idea into your life, you don't have to do it overnight, but you must start a trend. Don't go off M&M's cold turkey—or ever. It's the whole trajectory of your life that matters. Don't go on a twelve-week program that you believe will permanently solve all your problems. *There is no such program.* Don't drug yourself unnecessarily. It won't work.

Instead, start a trend. You may have a great couple of days followed by a total failure (in the form of a hot fudge sundae). *That's okay.* What's critical is that you've started a trend toward better living.

I see it all the time as a pastor—people who destroy their lives quickly and want to recover just as quickly. Life doesn't work that way. You can lose a fortune in a matter of minutes, but you probably won't get rich overnight. You can develop unhealthy habits quickly, but it's harder to regain your health in a hurry. Success takes a little while. You have to slowly incorporate a new approach.

There is a pragmatic side to this. As you read this book, you'll develop a specific, long-term plan that gives you a daily approach to eating and exercising. And there's only one thing to buy if you don't already have it: a good digital scale. If you can't afford one, save the money until you can. (Expect to spend at least $250.) You are going to set your life by this digital scale, so it needs to be accurate. And you'll love watching the numbers fall.

In the midst of the Jerusalem Diet plan, you can relax and enjoy life. If you love hot fudge sundaes, you can eat hot fudge sundaes. They're good for you! It is good to be able to kick back with family and friends and genuinely, happily enjoy something as wonderfully scrumptious as ooey-gooey hot fudge drizzled over rich vanilla ice cream.

With the Jerusalem Diet you can have that experience without guilt. Is it because I have some special product that makes hot fudge produce muscle rather than fat? No. It's because I think you shouldn't worry about the pleasure you get from hot fudge. It should be a sensible part of your life.

Look, I love Baskin-Robbins ice cream with a passion. I jokingly tell people that if I am going to die three years early because I eat Baskin-Robbins every week, then I'll go ahead and die three years early! Why live longer but without Baskin-Robbins?

Go easy. *Lighten up.* Don't be so hard on yourself. When you forgive yourself, it opens the door to change. It opens the door for the cravings and eating tendencies in your life to be adjusted.

To encourage you along the way, throughout the book I've inserted comments I've received from people like you who are already using the Jerusalem Diet. I think you'll find their insights helpful and their enthusiasm contagious.

This diet—yes, life itself—is a marathon, not a sprint. Read this book slowly and begin the program when you finish. Prepare to smile. Prepare to hope. Prepare to feel better. Prepare to improve the rest of your life.

Enjoy the Jerusalem Diet.

I Love Food!

I love food.

I love everything about food. I love the way it looks. I love the way it smells. I love thinking about it. I love buying it. I love cooking it. And of course I love eating it. I *love, love, love* eating it.

I love food so much that I sweat when I eat.

Maybe I love food because I was raised in a large family with lots of great food. Our meals were long and loud—especially loud. They were noisy affairs, with clanging pans, cracking ice-cube trays, clinking silverware, and lots of discussion—everyone telling stories, Mom bringing out more food and desserts, and Dad laughing at our stories and our smiles. It's no wonder to me that people who are heavy have a reputation for being happy. My family was proof positive that indulging in great meals can bring lots of joy.

The Haggard social life was formed around food. Marathon dinners were a family highlight (I've continued some of these traditions in my own family). I can still picture everyone sitting around piles of mashed potatoes and gravy, beef, chicken, loads of green beans, corn on the cob with warm butter melting down the sides, cold milk, iced tea, and pies, cobblers, and ice cream for dessert. Mom often thought she was making too much food, but in the end we'd be scraping the mashed potato bowl and competing for the last slice of cherry pie.

Because of those meals, which happened not just at Thanksgiving and Easter but every Sunday after church and many evenings during the week, I associate food with good conversation, laughter, and love. To this day, fried chicken, pot roast, and mashed potatoes and gravy are heaven for me! When I'm together with friends or family, we eat. It's a social ritual, and it's fun.

I love good food, and I also love what it creates. Food opens the door to gathering with good friends around the table. Such meals provide a kind of security. Food is deep, enriching conversation. Food is lighthearted story-telling. Food is laughter. Food is *so much fun.* Food, family, and friends—they go together.

The aroma of certain foods cooking reminds me of special people in my life. I know the smell of Grandma's house at Christmas and the smell of Mom's cooking in the kitchen. The aromas are symbolic as well as satisfying.

But food isn't just a heartwarming childhood memory. Food is a hobby. I love to snack. I eat while watching television. Nachos, fruit, candy, cookies, popcorn, or an orange—anything will do. I eat while working in the yard, taking breaks for sandwiches, an apple or an orange. I eat bananas while I read. I like to eat when I am in my office sitting around the conference table, working on projects with friends. And when there is a serious business meeting, we eat while we work. It helps all of us relax and enjoy the experience more. (I'm thinking about grabbing a snack right now!)

When my wife and I go out, we eat. When we have friends over, we eat. Chicken-salad sandwiches, broiled fish, grilled tenderloin, barbecued hamburgers, watermelon, nuts, iced tea, cookies, ice cream—they're all so incredibly great! There's nothing better than having good friends come over to eat slice after slice of pizza with ice-cold Mountain Dew or Coke.

Or, better yet, Jelly Bellies. Mmmmm, I love Jelly Bellies.

I keep a large bowl of Jelly Bellies in the center of my conference table right beside a bowl of nuts. They are both serious midday snacks, but Jelly Bellies have a special place in my heart. Why? Because they each have a unique flavor for only four calories a bean. Yes, it's true—just four calories for a tongue-tingling punch! My guess is that it takes just about that many calories to reach over and eat one, so it might be impossible to gain weight on Jelly Bellies. (Just hoping.)

Jelly Bellies are not casual food for me. They are serious business. I like the red ones best. My office staff buys them in jumbo-sized bags. They buy one bag of assorted flavors and another bag of all red. We mix them all in one bowl, but this way we are able to maintain a high red-to-nonred Jelly Belly ratio, which is very important for my emotional health. If I ever ran out of red Jelly Bellies before the end of the day, I might need therapy.

As I said, the Jelly Belly bowl sits in the middle of the conference table. Being a pastor, I have tons of meetings, and during each meeting I can enjoy a handful or two or three or four or five. Jelly Bellies make people feel good, and they cover for me when I can't think of anything to say in the meeting—my mouth is too full to talk.

Why do I go to hockey and baseball games? No question—because certain foods taste best in those settings. To me, hot dogs are only good at sporting events or on campouts. I'll take nachos anytime, and there's something about big pretzels with salt that makes a Coke or a Slurpee taste soooo good at a game. For me, the ticket price to a hockey, baseball, or basketball game is just a down payment on a pretzel and Coke—and a slice of pizza as well. (I love America!)

Camping is another activity that makes food taste better. Perfectly browned large marshmallows with chocolate and graham crackers—these things taste right only around a campfire. Mornings are great outdoors. I have a special way to prepare eggs, hash browns, and bacon that, I'm telling you, could be served in the finest restaurants.

Sometimes I go to a movie mostly to eat popcorn with extra popcorn salt so the drink tastes extra good. Why is popcorn better in a theater than anywhere else? And why do Slurpees taste best with salted popcorn?

Food and sports. Food and recreation. Food and family. Food and friends. Food, food, food!

Okay, I'm getting way too excited. Let me catch my breath.

When we enjoy food wisely, we will enjoy life. Food is the given. It's the wisely that is hard.

Ironically, I'm writing this chapter while staying at the King David Hotel in Jerusalem. I'm here as a guest of the Ministry of Tourism to meet with Israel's minister of finance, Benjamin Netanyahu, and prime minister, Ariel Sharon. In most of our meetings we have food. If we don't, the Israeli government takes us to a meal before or after the meeting. Why? Because they are wise! They know that meals make meetings better. Food provides the social setting necessary to visit without pressure. Food makes friends of strangers.

This is a great place to be writing about food. In this location, I'm near the Mount of *Olives,* the location of the Last *Supper.* I'm close to the place where Jesus asked his disciples to become *fishers* of men and first identified himself as the *Bread* of Life. And where people seeking God have celebrated many *feasts* of…well, you name it. You can't be Jewish, Christian, or Muslim without appreciating religious feasts. People of all faiths rejoice in food.

Now that I've been writing about food for a little while, I'm hungry. I just called room service. Today I am on target with my weight, so I can eat whatever I choose. If it was a Fat Day, I'd have to be more careful. I'll explain what all of this means in the next chapter.

Here in Jerusalem, there is a McDonald's down the road, but I decided to order room service instead. Don't get me wrong—I love McDonald's. I watched the documentary *Super Size Me* and craved a Big Mac afterward. That movie didn't discourage me; it just reminded me of McDonald's, which made me hungry. Not only do I like McDonald's, but KFC, Burger King, Taco Bell, Wendy's, Classic Drive-Thru Hamburgers (my favorite), and Carl's Jr. are always special treats. It's worth a trip to California just to get an In-and-Out double cheeseburger. I love these restaurants so much! My sister, Rachel, says that McDonald's french fries are one of the wonders of the world. The only reason I'm not going there now is that I'd have to put on my socks and shoes, and I'm too cozy to bother.

Ah…a knock at the hotel room door. Room service. A slender, black-haired Israeli guy just delivered a roast-beef sandwich with fries and a Coke. He did a good job. Lots of ketchup and plenty of napkins. I love that man!

(Pause in writing.)

Where was I? Hmmmm. Oh yeah. I love food.

By now you might be thinking you don't want to read this book since it's obviously written by a compulsive man expressing unrestrained admiration for foods that are dangerously tempting for you. Let me assure you—if you want a strict diet book with a photo of the perfect man on the cover or a diet book with pictures of an eighty-five-year-old woman who looks twenty-one, this is not the book for you. Or if you want a book that will point you to the one food that will transform you into a supermodel in one month, this book isn't what you're looking for.

I am not putting down those kinds of diet books. Many of them are helpful. I've read many of them and appreciated their tips. If I could do what they recommend for an extended period of time, I wouldn't need the Jerusalem Diet. If I could invest the time in exercising and eating according to their recommended plans, and if I had the money to buy the specialized products, I could probably get all the benefits promised.

But honestly, the demands of all these eating-exercising plans are too much for me. I'm busy living. I can't change my thinking patterns and lifestyle as quickly as some diet books require. They say eating no carbs or eating only carbs or doing daily abs workouts is easy, but it's not for me. Why?

I have a large family, which means hypercontrolling my diet and preparing specialized meals might inspire the first shots of a revolution.

I have a demanding and nontraditional job, which means a time-consuming exercise routine is very difficult to maintain.

I don't have much self-discipline. If interrogators threatened to withhold chocolate from me, I fear I might give up state secrets that would bring the end of freedom as we know it.

I like to eat.

And lastly, my knees hurt, and I'm tired after working all day.

Without these issues, I could do the good things recommended by some diet, exercise, and nutrition books. I believe all of them. I know I need good food, regular exercise, and supplements to improve my skin, cleanse my bowels, and extend my life. I believe it all. I want to do it all.

But I don't.

Because I can't.

I'm a loser. Who loves food.

I hope this dilemma does not apply to you, but for most of you, it does. If you love regular food but are willing to give it up while you choke down fiber, contort your body into bizarre positions, and avoid anything you can buy in the regular produce section of a grocery store, you'll do great without this book.

But if you like organic foods and take supplements, yet also have a hidden affection for the evil processed foods in which the capitalistic system has invested millions (no, billions) of dollars to make them taste *perfect,* then you will love this book.

A Balanced Diet (That Includes Food We Like)

This book is for people who love to eat. This book is for people who appreciate diet, exercise, and nutrition books but have a deep-rooted problem with their own humanity. This book is for people who want to be healthy but are not willing to give up their lives.

This book is for people who are willing to improve, but it's got to be easy. It's for people who like to smile. It's for people who are okay with looking the way they look while also aiming to improve their health and appearance. It's for people who eat ice cream in the dark. It's for people who sneak a Venti Mocha Frappuccino and then do penance for three days.

It's for people who live in perpetual guilt—or at least should live in perpetual guilt.

Okay, I've been munching on my room-service lunch as I've been writing, and now I am so full I can hardly sit up. Good thing it's an on-target day for me.

I wasn't kidding about loving Jelly Bellies and french fries. Of course I know if I eat those things in any way proportional to my affection for them, I won't feel very good. And they may kill me. I might even stop enjoying them so much, and I would really hate that.

So I've discovered a balance. I've discovered a way to enjoy life, enjoy food, be reasonable about my health, and at the same time maintain my work schedule and an energetic family and social life.

THE TRUTH ABOUT ME: DIETS WORK, I DON'T

I am not overweight, but I could be. Both my parents were well beyond a healthy weight. My dad died of a heart attack when he was fifty-eight. When my mom died, she had diabetes, arthritis, and numerous other diseases exacerbated by her obesity. If I want to improve my chances of keeping my health and living my full life span, I have to pay attention. But I'm weak. I'm undisciplined. I'm not the perfect man on the cover of *Men's Health*. I don't have time to live at the gym.

But after implementing the Jerusalem Diet, I'm not out of shape. According to my doctor, I'm a picture of health. Given my love of food, my enjoyment of sleep, and my fondness for lazy Saturdays lounging in pajamas all day, I could easily be in trouble. Without the ideas you'll find in this book, I might be obese.

I need a diet that is doable, not for some highly motivated guy who cares about the microbiology of digestion, but for me—an average guy wanting to live a good life. I need a plan I don't have to think about all the time. I need a plan I won't quit just because I drive past a Wendy's.

I was on the Atkins diet for a year—every day until noon. Why? Because I have many business lunches and meals with friends. It's too hard for a guy like me to ditch 90 percent of the carbs. I like bread. I also like pasta. I can live without them, but I can't live *well* without them.

I also failed at Atkins because of bedtime snacks. I'm like a ten-year-old— I have to snack before bedtime. Usually it's just a bowl of cereal, but sometimes I like yogurt or a toasted cheese sandwich or a plate of beanie weenies with bread and butter and a cold glass of milk. This really messes up the Atkins plan.

Atkins works. I don't.

South Beach works. I don't.

The Maker's Diet works. I don't.

When I hear the health-food crowd talk about tofu burgers and puréed yam soup and whole wheat udon, it makes my taste buds hide. I start thinking that an early death really might not be that bad after all. My taste buds scream, "We want *pleasure*!" And my intestines cry out, "We want to be clean but not *that* clean!"

I know all about making and breaking resolutions. I have an advanced education concerning commitment and failure. I'm a pastor. I teach people that the ancient scriptures tell them to be kind to one another, and they nod in agreement. Then, within a month, two of those who nodded are in my office talking about suing one another. I tell people that life will go better for them if they'll get up every morning and pray, and they are all for it. Some of them will actually do it, some never will, and most will try and stop and try and stop and try and stop. People are people. We are the problem.

It's the same with diet and health. We are the problem. Throw a rock and you'll hit a diet book that would really help you. Spend ten minutes on Google, and you'll have a wealth of nutrition information to help shape your eating habits. You can get the facts, but you might not be able to apply them. Those red Jelly Bellies taste too good. (Who makes Jelly Bellies, anyway? They should win a Nobel Prize for making a product that good!) Or, if Jelly Bellies don't do it for you, name your weakness. Ice cream? Soda? French fries? Caramel corn? Chocolate?

Yeah, thanks to loads of diet-and-nutrition guides, we know how to solve the problem of our eating habits. But we probably won't. Most of the solutions are too dramatic. Surgery might help, but it hurts. Ow! And for me, most diets ask too much. They change our lifestyles 100 percent too quickly, and we don't have the time, patience, or willpower for 100 percent change. So we lose weight and gain weight; we exercise every day and then don't hit the gym for a month; we eat proteins and veggies and then buy stock in Häagen-Dazs.

Does any of this sound familiar to you? I have a solution.

CHAPTER 2

"My Pants Are Too Tight!" ...A Diet Discovery

N ow I'm back in Colorado Springs in my backyard on a seventy-nine-degree, sunny Friday afternoon. The sky is an incredible, brilliant blue with one beautiful puffy white cloud. The grass is green and perfectly groomed. The flowers around the trees are in full bloom, and the crystal-clear water in the pool is a refreshing eighty-six degrees. My eleven-year-old son, Elliott, and his buddy Josiah are splashing around in the water. Music is playing in the background, combining with the sound of a gentle breeze blowing through the trees.

I feel great. How did life get this good?

This morning when I woke up, my wife, Gayle, brought me a bowl of raspberries while I was reading the paper and working on a few e-mails in bed. The raspberries were fantastic. I got up and took my vitamins (fish oil for my whole body, a multivitamin to fill in the gaps, glucosamine and chondroitin for my joints, lutein and beta carotene for my eyes, and fiber for...my personal life). I ate an apple and drank a large glass of water.

At noon, Gayle and I went to a friend's home for lunch. For an appetizer we had half a tomato with salmon, dressed with a delicious sauce on a bed of carrot and Waldorf salad. For our entrée, we dined on four ounces of lean lamb with sliced sweet potato, rice, and a vegetable dish served with whole-wheat pita bread to dip into olive oil and chopped olives. Man, this meal was delicious!

As I write this, it's 3:21 in the afternoon. I'm drinking a refreshing Mountain Dew. At 7:00 p.m. I'm scheduled to go to the Boulder Street Church downtown to perform a wedding for some good friends. Then I'll come home and share a thin-crust mushroom-and-sausage pizza and a hand-tossed supreme pizza with my family before we all go to bed.

Does it sound like my life revolves around food? Well, sort of! However, I've not given you this schedule because I'm self-absorbed and think you are interested in the details of my life. I gave it to you as an example. Remember, I'm a forty-nine-year-old guy with a busy life, and I have an idea about how to stay healthy without being consumed in the minutiae that is required by some health experts.

Note that during the first half of the day, I ate *real* food—good-for-you, nutritious food. Then, without guilt or the prospect of getting fat, I plunged into the debauchery of a cold Mountain Dew poured over crushed ice in a big glass.

After reading the first chapter, you might think I'm the worst person in the world to give counsel on health and diet. True enough. I don't claim to be an expert on the subject. I just know that I love food, but I also have a system that keeps me healthy and relatively fit. Granted, I like joking around with this subject, but I do know that diet, rest, exercise, and a positive mental attitude are very important.

I will never minimize the importance of proper nutrition and exercise. If you are overweight, your feet and knees are bearing unnecessary strain. You have a greater likelihood of developing a variety of illnesses, such as heart disease, cancer, arthritis, and diabetes. In the end, you may die sooner than you should. Even if you are not overweight, if you have very unhealthy eating habits and never exercise, you could be in trouble.

But I believe in an attitude toward diet and exercise that works for common people. I believe in helping you laugh a little and approach the subject with a smile instead of the usual agony that comes with reading another diet book.

I believe in basic plumb lines and small goals but also in grand indulgences and lots of joy. In this book you'll see how you can lose weight slowly and effectively and how you can do it in a context of happiness and excitement.

If you'll laugh with me and begin enjoying life, it will be easier for you to achieve your ideal weight. Let me emphasize: I'm no doctor or nutritionist. But I do pastor a church of eleven thousand people, and I am in the business of helping people live the life that God designed for them. Because of that, I am responsible for observing life closely and coming up with advice that helps all of us.

MOUNTAIN DEW DAYS

Many diets encourage people to follow a plan so they can lose hundreds of pounds in a short time and look as if they have been disciplined and fit all their lives. Well, I'm of the persuasion that if we take the pills, buy the supplements, exercise for an hour and a half a day, and eat like rabbits, it might be better just to go ahead and die.

I have friends who are so diet conscious that they have lost their social lives. They can't go to friends' homes or social events, because they can't eat anything that is served. They have specialized diets. And they smell bad. Yes, that's right. They think it's good, but because they are always "detoxifying," they stink. They have body odor, bad breath, and awful-looking skin. I think they need a pizza.

I would rather die early than do what they are doing. But I want to live well. That's why I'm drinking a Mountain Dew.

Why Mountain Dew? It's a fine, healthy drink. (Note: This is my sense of humor. If you are too seriously engaged with this topic, skip this paragraph.) Oh yes, Mountain Dew! The first ingredient is water, which is so good for us. The second ingredient is corn syrup. Corn! A vegetable—a staple of American life. The third ingredient is orange juice. Water, corn, and orange juice—what could be better? I'm shocked that no one has ever written a book called *The Mountain Dew Diet*.

Okay, I know that Mountain Dew is not on the list of healthy drinks. But Mountain Dew is one of the beverages that make a sunny afternoon special. To drink water would be fine, but to sit out here in my backyard with water might make the blue sky gray, the grass brown, and the pool water cold. Nope, this setting requires a Mountain Dew. And that's okay.

❧

Here I am, writing again. A day has passed, and I'm in my backyard again.

You'll never believe what's happening!

NBC News is doing a documentary on evangelicals, so they wanted some shots of me sitting in the backyard with my family and doing my work. The NBC crew has their camera pointed at me as I type! I wonder, *How could this be interesting to anyone? Are twenty-four-hour news outlets this desperate for content?* Well, now you know—if you ever see the documentary—that the shot of me supposedly working on a sermon or a position paper on some topic of current interest was actually just me writing about how much I love Mountain Dew!

Okay, they got what they want. Now let me tell you the story of the Jerusalem Diet.

MY PANTS WERE TOO TIGHT

It was 1998. I was in Jerusalem, touring Israel with a group. I was having a great time seeing the world with some of my best friends.

Then I realized I was fat.

One morning I got up, showered, and started getting dressed. My pants didn't quite fit. Too snug. Not baggy and comfortable. Not relaxed. I hated the feeling.

I realized that I'd been sucking in my belly to fasten my pants for some time, but I was getting larger and larger. So I'd bought bigger pants every couple of months, mostly without thinking about it much. But here, in Jerusalem, it dawned on me. *I'm a fat guy. I'm getting ugly. My body is changing. I look better in clothes than I do naked! I'm in trouble.*

I switched to another pair of pants. Nope, too tight. Another pair. Those didn't fit, either.

Uh-oh.

All my pants were too tight. I had just entered the baggy-sweat-suit stage. Sucking in my gut wasn't going to work anymore. I was in trouble. I looked in the mirror. Did my T-shirt always look this small?

I had been gaining notches on my belt for months, but I was too busy, too lazy to worry about it. My wife had been kind enough not to say anything. But now I was in crisis. I couldn't ignore reality. It was happening to me. I was getting fat.

I let myself be bummed for an hour, but I knew if I dwelled on this, I'd beat myself up. And probably beat up a few members of my staff too. Instead, I began to consider what to do about my swelling size. Some thoughts came.

Everything I'd read on health mentioned the importance of fruits, vegetables, and nuts. No way was I ready to become a vegetarian, but I wondered what would happen if I limited my eating, *just for one day,* to fruits, vegetables, and nuts. I knew I wouldn't want to keep that limitation for long, but for one day it sounded great. I felt so lazy and fat—I had to do *something*. I wanted to kick-start my body toward better health. The adventure factor alone would get me through one day, right? I wasn't sure it would help, but I figured it couldn't hurt, and if I felt a little better about myself, it would be worth it. I decided to give it a shot.

When I went to breakfast, I realized my plan was going to be easy because I was in the Middle East. The table was stocked with fruits, vegetables, and a concoction of nuts and seeds, so I added seeds to my list of what was acceptable. I went the rest of the day eating only those four types of foods.

Remarkably, I never got hungry all day. Everywhere we went, fruits, vegetables, nuts, or seeds were available, so no one noticed I was eating differently. I didn't say anything to anyone and ate to my satisfaction. I noticed that my appetite was less. When I wanted to nibble, I grabbed a handful of nuts. Rather than drinking soft drinks, I drank only water. I felt great.

Just before dinner our team had a free hour, so I went back to the hotel and worked out. I wasn't able to run very long, swim very far, or lift much weight, but I did what I could for about an hour.

That night when I lay down in bed, I felt fit. I felt good. I felt satisfied. I was amazed. I was not as tired as normal and stayed up awhile longer before hitting the bed.

The next morning—I know this sounds crazy, but it's true—my clothes felt better on me. My body had reacted quickly to my one-day diet. I'm not saying my waist size shrank or the love handles magically disappeared, but I felt better. My clothes *looked* like they fit better, and I certainly felt good about the way I was eating.

The Jerusalem Diet was born.

CHAPTER 3

The Jerusalem Diet:
Secret, Simple, and Flexible

I woke up fat this morning. You know the feeling. You can see it coming the night before.

Yesterday was a great day. I was scheduled to do a one-hour interview with Tom Brokaw from NBC. The network called and expanded the schedule, and we ended up spending more than two hours together. I think the interview went very well. There is no way to tell for sure, though, until the editing is done. But I felt great.

As a result, I was excited last evening, so at 8:30 I got the kids and called the Parsleys—Ross, the church's associate pastor, his wife, Aimee, and their four kids—and we all went to the Black-Eyed Pea restaurant. I hadn't been there for years, but I was hungry for meat loaf, mashed potatoes, corn, and a Coke. We stayed until 11:00. We came home, and I went to bed feeling as satisfied as a cat purring in front of a stove on a winter day. I slept very soundly.

But, oh, this morning was terrible. I knew it would be a Fat Day, which means I'm at least one pound over my target weight. (*Fat Day? Target weight?* I'll explain in a minute.) I was right. After I woke up and used the bathroom, I weighed myself as usual. I have a nice digital scale that is very accurate. I stepped on and saw the bad news—yup, I was a pound heavy for the day.

Because it was a Fat Day, I had to limit my diet to fruits, vegetables, nuts, and seeds. I drank only water and exercised for one hour.

For breakfast, after taking my vitamins with water, I had a bowl of cherries.

After eating breakfast, I went to the track and ran three miles. That took about thirty minutes. Then I got into the pool and swam for thirty minutes.

For lunch I had a salad.

During the day I munched on trail mix, apples, and a banana.

At suppertime, I wasn't very hungry, so I didn't eat. Later I snacked on a couple of tangerines before I went to bed.

Tomorrow when I wake up, I'll be on or under my target weight.

That's it. You've just learned the basics of the Jerusalem Diet. It's easy. You don't have to commit to six weeks, six months, or six years of a particular eating pattern. People don't have to know you are "doing the Jerusalem Diet." You control your weight and address your overall health by being disciplined for one day.

This works for me. I can control what I eat and do for a day, but two days is too much. A week, no way. A month, forget it.

You already know that a one-day adjustment won't give you the body of an Olympic gymnast. But a one-day success will have a moderate, immediate, and definite impact on your well-being. Even if you feel your body does not change much, getting through a day of fruits, vegetables, nuts, seeds, water, and an hour of exercise is a sign that you are headed in the right direction. You can build on that one day and transform your life.

During the years I've used the Jerusalem Diet, I've never committed to anything beyond one day. On Fat Days, as I eat fruits, vegetables, nuts, and seeds—and enjoy water and an hour of exercise—I don't have to think, *Oh, great, no Jelly Bellies for a month.* Instead, I think, *Was eating all of those Jelly Bellies yesterday worth this? If I hadn't eaten them, I wouldn't be having a Fat Day today, and I could eat a few. Now I have to wait until tomorrow.*

I remember days when I ran around the track thinking, *Was the Mountain Dew worth this?* Or, *If I hadn't eaten those nachos last night, I would be on target today, and I wouldn't have to do this.* As you know, you don't stop thinking while exercising. When I exercise on my Fat Days, I think about the snacks I ate the day before and wonder if they were worth it. I think about the fact that there is nothing in my body that I didn't eat. I put those M&M's in there of my own free will. No one forced that Coke down my throat. I have no one to blame but myself. So while running, I think about limiting the types of food I'll eat tomorrow to avoid having another Fat Day soon.

But enough of this reflection about my experiences. It's time for a quick summary of the Jerusalem Diet.

THE JERUSALEM DIET IN A NUTSHELL

If you read the rest of this chapter carefully, the sun will shine for you again. You'll learn how to improve your health and life. You'll have hope, perspective, and excitement about the future. And you'll know how to start today.

Here is what you need to do:

1. *Buy an accurate digital scale.* If possible, test the scale before you purchase it by stepping onto it a few times to ensure it shows your weight the same—repeatedly. This is the only thing you absolutely have to buy; everything else (which is to say, food) is probably already in your pantry and fridge. You will notice, however, that you will need more fruits, vegetables, nuts, and seeds for the days you are overweight. On other days you will find yourself increasingly wanting healthier foods, and you may enjoy exploring other health and exercise products. But you don't have to buy anything except a good digital scale.

2. *Determine your ideal weight.* No ideal weight chart is perfect. In fact, I can't find one that I really like. None of them seem to provide

consistent, reliable figures on my weight. So let me recommend that you do what I do: find several Web sites that will calculate it more specifically for you. (If you don't have Internet access, stop at your local library or call a friend who can help.) I just paused in my writing, went to Google on the Internet, and typed in "ideal weight." A long list of sites came up. I went to four of them, entered my information, and came up with my ideal weight. I'm forty-nine years old, five feet eleven, with a medium build. My ideal weight is 172 pounds. That's my plumb line for health.

3. *Take a calendar and mark your weight on today's date.* Then go forward one week and mark one pound less. Do that for as many weeks as it takes to reach your ideal weight. (Stop and reread this and think about it until you understand it.) Do it one pound, one week at a time. This is important. If you lose weight faster than this, your body will fight you. You'll look too different too quickly. Your body may not adjust as you lose weight, and your friends will notice. *Don't do it.* Instead, slowly and steadily lose weight so that your friends don't notice. Let them develop the vague notion that you are looking and feeling better. In time, they'll be shocked at how different you look. Your body will have time to adjust if you lose at the one-pound-a-week rate, and your mind and emotions will have time to adjust to an improved diet and lifestyle of exercise. It may have taken years to get into your present shape. Now, be sensible. As you start the process of reclaiming the best body you can get, let time be your friend, not your enemy. You have your whole life to live.

4. *Weigh yourself each day at the same time.* This is crucial—it'll remind you every day where you are in your process. I weigh myself when I get up in the morning, immediately after using the rest room. I have a calendar in my bathroom that I write my daily weight on. If

I'm over my target weight, I call that a Fat Day. If I'm exactly at my target weight, I can eat what I want, but I know I have to be careful, or I'll have a Fat Day the next day. If I'm under a pound or two, Baskin-Robbins, here I come! *If you are at or below your target weight* on any particular day, eat what you like and exercise if you want to. In time, you'll learn to work with your temptations, habits, styles, tastes, schedule, and bodily responses to the decisions you make. You'll learn what you can get away with and what you can't. You'll learn to break your own rules when you want to and to be more strict when you need to. *If you are over your target weight,* for one day eat only fruits, vegetables, nuts, and seeds. Drink only water. Exercise for one hour. Later I'll explain why fruits, vegetables, nuts, seeds, water, and exercise are the winning combination.

Yes, it's that simple. When I'm on target for the day, I eat whatever I want. That's how it is most of the time. But if I indulge too much and/or exercise too little, I'll have a Fat Day. On those days, though, I don't have to consult one recipe. I don't have to look for special foods. All I have to do is eat real food for a day. I can go about my business, and often people don't even notice I'm eating differently than usual.

When I follow this system, I can lose one pound per week with no problem. Actually, I can lose one pound per day, but as I said (and will explain more later), it is not good to lose too much weight too quickly. So having a Fat Day means losing one pound. At that point, I have met my weight-loss goal for the week. If I happen to go over my target weight again during the week, I have another Fat Day. But most of the time, one day of fruits, vegetables, nuts, seeds, water, and an hour of exercise will mean losing one pound, meeting my target weight for the week, and steadily progressing toward my ideal weight.

I should say here that I prefer using ideal weight rather than body-mass index (BMI) or body-fat percentage because ideal weight is easy to check every day. Other people will say you need to go by BMI (which is also easy to check online), waist size, or some other indicator. That's fine. But checking your weight every day is as easy as stepping on a scale. I appreciate that convenience and find that it gives me the motivation I need to try to be fit.

I can see right now that this approach will probably not help my bank account much. I'm not selling you any specialized supplements. I don't have any medical or exercise equipment to market. I just want you to buy real foods and eat them. I want you to exercise and use whatever supplements and other diet programs you enjoy. If you do this, you'll be very satisfied.

This approach works for me. Why? Because I'm not interested in being consumed by a diet. I don't want a specialized diet that redefines my whole life. I just want a plan that keeps me from killing myself with the wrong kinds of food but still allows me to eat what I like. I want a plan that will help me grow toward healthy living without implicating everyone around me and forcing them into my system.

I think this diet will work for you, too. It's secret, simple, and flexible—all attributes of a diet you can use for the rest of your life.

THE SECRET DIET

I don't wear my eating habits on my sleeve. I like to be thoughtful and careful about meals and snacking, but I also like to indulge. So I don't want to feel as though I'm under surveillance.

Because their restrictions were so severe, some of the diets I tried in the past virtually required me to make a public service announcement:

Attention: Ted Haggard Is Now Officially on an All-Grapefruit Diet.
Any Offerings of Non-Grapefruit Items Will Be Rejected. Please
Respect Ted's Dieting Privileges. No Good Food, Not Even Grapefruit-
Flavored Jelly Bellies, Should Be Offered Until Further Notice.

Most of the time I don't want my diet to be anyone else's business. My wife knows, but no one else needs to know.

Part of the reason this is important is that it keeps other people from feeling pressured by my eating habits. Before long, Gayle and I will be invited to a dinner, and we'll be served, say, pan-seared salmon with herbed potatoes. If I were on a regular, restrictive diet, I'd have to make a big show of my newfound distaste for carbohydrates: "No potatoes for me, please! Oh, those look great, but no sirree! It's just not worth those extra carbs. Yep, they turn right to fat, you know. But help yourself!"

What if the person serving me dinner is fifty pounds heavier than I am? How will that make him feel? I want to lose weight, but I don't want to be a jerk about it.

I also don't want to have to deal with the shame of failure. Mind you, as a pastor, I understand the upside of shame. When people come to my office to report all kinds of bad things they want to do, or have done, or that their "friends" have done, I'm glad their shame motivated them to talk about it. And I, too, want to feel shame when I should feel shame. Shame can keep me safe. But I don't want to go seeking shame where I don't have to. I want to enjoy life, and I want to enjoy food. I *love* food. Why would I want to feel shameful eating it?

I've been in people's homes or out to eat on a Fat Day, and I've had meat on my salad or eaten whatever I needed to eat in order to be polite. But because it's a Fat Day, I don't overeat. And as soon as I'm in a situation where I can control my nutrition decisions again, I go back on the plan.

Now, guess what? I can't remember one day when "blowing my diet" on a Fat Day kept me from being back on weight the next day. The only thing that has kept me from correcting in one day is if I just eat, eat, eat and totally disregard the Jerusalem Diet. Then the pounds add up.

Since this plan is inconspicuous, I don't have to worry about public opinion. I lost weight as soon as I began this diet, but if I hadn't, no one would have known. As I dropped the pounds slowly over a reasonable period of time, the weeks turned into months, and I finally heard those wonderful, wonderful words: "Ted, have you lost weight?"

That's a great bonus—when people eventually notice and compliment your appearance. But in the meantime, there are two major benefits to keeping a diet secret:

1. If no one knows about my diet, then I can't make anyone else feel guilty.
2. If no one knows about my diet, then no one can make me feel guilty.

A guilt-free diet? Imagine that!

The Simple Diet

I also need my diet to be easy. For me, simplicity is a virtue. I want things to be painless, which makes them more doable.

I want a diet that respects my right to be lazy.

My one-day diet adjustment requires almost no thinking at all. Consider the circumstances of its inauguration during my trip in Jerusalem: The idea occurred to me in the morning, and I was able to follow it all day with zero preparation, zero planning, and zero pain. I didn't prepare any special foods. I didn't buy a single ounce of supernutrient product. I just went about my business and ate what was available as long as it was a fruit, vegetable, nut, or seed.

When I exercised that first day on the diet, I made it a goal to continue for sixty minutes. I wasn't severe about this—I didn't start my stopwatch and check my heart rate or maintain any sort of consistency during that time. I walked on the treadmill for several minutes, then jogged. I hopped on a couple of the weight machines for a few sets, then cooled off by jumping into the pool where I swam a few laps. Before I knew it, an hour had passed, and I went back to my hotel room.

I knew that if I stuck to this program every single day—fruits, vegetables, nuts, seeds, water, and exercise—I could probably lose all my unwanted weight in a month. But did I really want to do that? Nah. It was fun for a day, but a month of it might have made me very, very miserable.

Between fun and misery, I choose fun.

I like nuts and seeds, but I don't want to eat like a bird all the time. I love jogging, but I rarely have a chance to pound the pavement for five miles a day. No, one day is about all I can take.

A one-day diet. A doable diet. A diet that requires very little effort on my part. Imagine that.

THE FLEXIBLE DIET

During that first Fat Day in Jerusalem, I loved the adventure factor of my one-day diet. I felt as if I had been on a little mission all day. The secrecy element was a big part of it—no one ever suspected that I was eating differently. (Because all my pants were too tight, they might have *wanted* me to eat differently, but I didn't want to give them the satisfaction of knowing that I was trying!) I watched people gobble down sweet rolls at breakfast, greasy sandwiches at lunch, and snack after snack in the afternoon, secretly knowing all the while that I was avoiding such things—just for that day.

But I was traveling in Israel and was fortunate that we visited places where fruits, vegetables, nuts, and seeds were readily available. I took a bag of trail mix as we traveled, rather than a candy bar. I drank water rather than soda. It was easy. The same would have been true back home in Colorado; just about any restaurant would have given me a choice of meatless salads or other entrées that let me stay on my one-day diet.

But what if at lunchtime on my one-day diet, I had been with people who *just had* to go to a burger joint and the only options were a cheeseburger or a bacon burger? As I've mentioned, I had already decided what I would do: I would simply break my diet, enjoy a reasonable amount of food, and try to keep it from pushing me into another Fat Day tomorrow.

When the choice is maintaining the diet or being free to eat what's available, I eat what's available in smaller portions. What's wrong with that? My overall diet plan isn't going anywhere, and as long as I am on a general trend toward healthiness, then the diet should allow for the fluctuations of my life.

A diet that adapts to my lifestyle, my schedule. A diet that I can change on the fly. Imagine that.

Let me say a little more about the flexibility factor, because it's a core value of the Jerusalem Diet. As I've been working on this book, several people who have heard me give talks on a healthy lifestyle have sent me testimonials of their experiences with the Jerusalem Diet. (You'll see some of these stories throughout this book.) All their experiences are encouraging; they report gradual but continual weight loss and increased time devoted to exercise. More important, they report a newfound sense of hope, a sharpened perspective on nutrition and health, and a new attitude about exercise.

But my favorite aspect of these testimonies is that when they describe the Jerusalem Diet, they describe individual experiences. One person reported discovering that a one-hour jog was perfect for him. Another said that spending eight minutes a day on her bicycle has been a major achievement. Another hasn't had time to exercise at all but has at least switched M&M's with almonds on her desk at work—and feels great about that decision. I love hearing about these small but important changes.

The Jerusalem Diet is a fill-in-the-blank diet. It's adaptable. It nudges you in the right direction. Take it and run with it.

"But I'm a Hundred Pounds Too Heavy!"

Back in Jerusalem, I had so enjoyed my one-day adjustment that I devised the little plan I've just outlined. Once I determined my ideal weight, I set a long-term goal to achieve that weight. I wasn't interested in dropping pounds overnight, mostly because I didn't want to have to change my eating habits or lifestyle all that much. Lose a pound a week—that seemed doable.

I found out what I weighed, found out what I wanted to weigh, and discovered a twenty-three pound difference. At a loss of one pound per week, it would take me about half a year to get to my ideal weight. To some people, that might seem like an eternity. To me, it seemed like a chance to diet successfully. I wouldn't be rushing to health. It wouldn't shock my body, my family, my friends, or my lifestyle. It would give me time. I would gradually reach my goal.

I know several people who had fifty, seventy-five, or a hundred pounds to lose when they began this diet. The amount doesn't matter, and the time line doesn't matter. If you are a hundred pounds overweight, then you can know that in two years you'll look and feel much better than you do now. Two years is not that long a time. And it will feel like the blink of an eye—especially if you improve your health for the rest of your life.

I'll say more about this in the "Change Your Life...Slowly" chapter, but let me mention that I am an advocate of gradual change. Our lives don't usually change by fits and starts; they change over time. Very few people become financially stable overnight. Most spend several years getting their finances in order, saving and investing a few dollars at a time. This isn't a problem; it's good for us to make these long-term commitments and to give ourselves space for a prolonged process. We need time to fail a little, adjust things, fail some more, adjust a little more, and so on, until we arrive at success.

So I grabbed a calendar. I counted out twenty-three weeks and wrote down the target weight that I wanted to reach for each week. Every week was one pound less than the previous week. One week back, one pound less. And so on, until I reached my ideal week and weight.

Now I had a *target weight* for each week leading up to my *ideal weight.* As I've said, I decided that I would get up every morning and weigh myself. If I was already at or below my target weight for that week, I would eat whatever I wanted that day. If I was above my target weight, then I would do the Jerusalem Diet that day, eating only fruits, vegetables, nuts, and seeds—plus drinking only water and exercising for one hour. The next morning I would be at or below my target weight. If not, I would do the Jerusalem Diet again. If I was on target, I would eat as I pleased.

If I had to go without Jelly Bellies, it would only be for one day—maybe two.

This seemed reasonable to me. I liked having six months. Moreover, I liked the *attitude* of the diet. I liked that I could live a normal life within it.

So—a one-day diet. That's the overall message. Stay on the plan, and it will produce for you. One day. That's all you have to do. One day.

Tomorrow you can eat cheese enchiladas. Tomorrow. Only one sleep away.

CHAPTER 4

All Diets Work
(but None Work for Me)

Today is not a Fat Day.

I got up this morning and, after going to the bathroom, weighed myself. I was a pound under my target weight. Even though I could have had whatever I wanted for breakfast, since I've been reading materials on diet, nutrition, and exercise, I actually wanted fresh tomato juice. So I took my vitamins with a large glass of water and then put one cup of water and three tomatoes into my blender. I blended them for thirty seconds, then I drank a full glass of juice. It tasted fantastic.

I went through the morning feeling great—full and optimistic.

Lunchtime came. I went with some friends to Pizza Hut but wasn't hungry. I had two small slices of pizza and a glass of Pepsi. That's all it took—I felt full.

I went all afternoon without being hungry.

This evening I wasn't hungry, but because I knew I needed to eat something and wanted to dine with the family, I had a cheese sandwich with chips and tea.

Now it's 11:14 p.m., and I'm up writing. I have popcorn and a glass of orange juice. I'm not really hungry. I'm just snacking as I write. I know I won't have a Fat Day tomorrow. Truthfully, I've been satiated most of the day because of my tomato-juice breakfast. You see tomatoes are a "superfood." Recently I learned of a group of foods that offer superb health benefits. These superfoods are described in detail in an intriguing book by Dr. Steven Pratt and Kathy Matthews entitled *Superfoods Rx: Fourteen Foods That Will Change Your Life*. (In addition to tomatoes, the superfoods are beans, blueberries, broccoli, oats, oranges, pumpkin, wild salmon, soy, spinach, green tea, black tea, turkey, and walnuts.)[1]

Obviously, this list of superfoods helped me. So did information from Dr. Atkins and every other nutritionist or dietitian I've read. They all helped shape the decisions I make daily about what goes into my body.

Take tonight, for instance. When I decided to get out of bed to come down and write this chapter, I was hungry for cinnamon rolls! I'm not having a Fat Day, so it's okay for me to have at least one of these big rolls with icing. I could have done it with no guilt. But once downstairs, I thought about the risk of having a Fat Day tomorrow and decided to have some popcorn instead. As I was walking into the garage to get a Coke with lime to drink with my popcorn, I thought about orange juice. That sounded better. I typically prefer making fresh orange juice, but tonight, to avoid the mess and the noise since my family is asleep, I poured a big glass of Tropicana Pure Premium Orange Juice fortified with calcium and vitamin D.

See the transformation? I'm being nudged in the right direction. I know, I know. Some readers are thinking that popcorn is bad carbs and that pre-prepared orange juice is dead. True. But popcorn is better than cinnamon rolls, and pre-prepared orange juice is better for me than soda. If you work for Coke, don't get yourself all in a dither. I'm not saying I'll never drink another Coke. I love Coke and may have one tomorrow. And I'm not a doctor or a nutritionist. I can't explain the science of why orange juice is better for me than Coke. But I've read that repeatedly, and I trust it is true.

The point is that I am gradually getting better, one pound at a time, one idea at a time, one victory over temptation at a time.

This is why the Jerusalem Diet will work for you. On this plan, you can utilize the knowledge of everything you learn, and you'll be on a slow, easy transition that will get your weight under control. You'll see results, slowly and steadily, and be able to enjoy your friends and food in the process.

EATING BETTER IN SPITE OF MYSELF

My problem with thinking about diets all the time, as I've been doing since I started writing this book, is that it makes me hungry.

Twice in the last week my editor called to discuss the manuscript. "What are you doing now?" he asked. "Is this a good time to go over the diet book?"

Both times I was out to eat or in a meeting where there was lots of food. I'm so embarrassed. I'm supposed to be the diet guy right now, and I'm loving my social and family times with food.

Both days, though, I was under my target weight for the day, so theoretically, it didn't matter in the grand Jerusalem Diet scheme. I was free to splurge. But of course, when I'm being really good, I don't eat as much junk even during on-target days. The stuff is bad for me. I know it. You can hardly be a citizen of the United States of America today and not know how much poison you're putting into your system every time you step outside your house. Newspapers and magazines are filled with reports on dangerous pesticides, poorly maintained slaughterhouses, and genetically modified produce. The Morgan Spurlocks *(Super Size Me)* and Eric Schlossers *(Fast Food Nation)* of the world do a fine job of filling in the dirty details of those reports.

Last night Gayle and I went shopping. Since I've been on the Jerusalem Diet, the produce department of our grocery story has become our favorite place to shop. When I see tomatoes (which I don't like to eat but I do like to drink), I always buy some. When I see walnuts, oranges, kiwis, bananas, clementines, blueberries, raspberries, cherries, nuts, and yogurt, I buy them. The difference, though, is that I'll buy a hearty granola for the days when I want it and Corn Pops for the occasional nights when I want something a little more fun.

As I am getting older and gaining more knowledge, I drink fewer caffeinated drinks and more drinks that are closer to pure water. Most of us are eating more food that is alive and less that is processed, and we exercise more, knowing that even when we eat poorly, if we're fit, the food that used to make us fat won't have quite the same effect.

I don't suffer from a lack of knowledge. I do, however, from time to time suffer from a lack of self-control. My affection for Jelly Bellies, Krispy Kreme doughnuts, and cheeseburgers is, no doubt, diminishing, but it still sometimes overwhelms my knowledge of how those foods make me feel. Being a big believer in free markets, I love to enjoy the advantages of an advanced marketplace with all its variety, opportunity, and affordability. Sometimes, even when I don't want a Krispy Kreme, I feel like picking up a dozen doughnuts as a matter of principle!

It's been worse since beginning this diet book, because I keep writing about all the things I shouldn't eat, which makes me think about the things I shouldn't eat, which makes me hungry for those things.

Why do we think that if we launch into a diet plan that requires us to think about our weight, our body, and food all day, every day, we'll end up fit? It seldom works, at least for people like me.

Instead, I need a plan that doesn't require so much of my attention. I love food, and I want a healthy life. Oh my, is there any hope for me?

The Bathroom Scale Monitor

Normally, when I'm not writing a diet book, when I'm not trying to think like a health advisor, when the thoughts of delicious root beer or rocky road ice cream aren't breathing down my neck, I am able to keep my divergences to a minimum because of one simple thing: the bathroom scale.

Because of the Jerusalem Diet, I know I am going to weigh myself the next day. The temptation to dive into a basket of fries is strong, but the number that stares up at me from the bathroom scale is stronger. Whatever I eat today will affect what I see on the scale readout tomorrow. (Okay, I'm dumping the rest of the popcorn in the trash and am finished with the orange juice for tonight. I'm convinced. I'm stuffed. I don't need to eat this way at this time of night.) Remember, on the Jerusalem Diet if you are at or below your target weight, you are free. You can do whatever you like—eat what you want and exercise if you want to. But understand: you are going to have to weigh yourself the next day.

So whenever the food cravings settle in (and some days they don't at all, especially if I've been eating healthy foods; on other days, little slip-ups have a snowball effect), I try to remember that in a few short hours I will step onto the scale and have to face facts. The number could climb, and if it does, I can look forward to a day of fruits, vegetables, nuts, and seeds.

Before I discovered this plan, I liked going to bed at night with a full stomach. I thought it would help me sleep. But after finding this plan and seeing the negative results of eating a lot of food just before bedtime, I avoided anything substantive after 7:00 p.m. I might eat yogurt or something like that, but I wouldn't be stuffed when I went to bed. When I go to sleep more empty, I almost always wake up at or below my target weight.

I love the way good food affects me. At times I talk myself into some decadence by deciding that I could use a day of eating like a rabbit, so a bowl of ice cream is worth it. And when this happens, I don't feel guilty. But as much as I enjoy my fruits, vegetables, nuts, seeds, water, and exercise days, it's more fun to choose what I want to eat all day. Many days I stick with veggies even though I'm on target with my weight, and some days I run three to six miles whether I'm over my target or not. But I'd rather have the option to do what I want, so the motivation to be on target is strong.

A Little Bit of Resentment Goes a Long Way

At times I have been just two-tenths of a pound over my target weight. Two-tenths of a pound! I know this because I have a digital scale. But I've pushed through my reluctance and stuck with fruits, vegetables, nuts, seeds, water, and an hour of exercise. As I'm on my third mile on the treadmill, huffing and puffing, I'm thinking, "I just *know* it was Taco Bell that put me over! It wasn't worth it."

Believe it or not, after a few days like this, I began to develop a little resentment toward too much junk food. Don't get me wrong—I still love the stuff. But I resent it too. I love to drink Mountain Dew, but I also have a little bit of hatred for this drink I love so much. And that little bit of hatred goes a long way. It doesn't mean I'll never drink Mountain Dew again; it just means I need to be careful, because the next morning I'll weigh myself again, and the number I see will determine my day for me. I'd rather determine the day for myself.

The Jerusalem Diet is training me.

These experiences of being over target and suffering the consequences are very valuable. I think they are what makes the Jerusalem Diet work for so many people—it's like a flexible, enjoyable system of trial and error. You have a goal, and when you don't meet that goal, you can take twenty-four hours to get it right, but in a relatively easy, enjoyable, and healthy way. And the whole attitude requires flexibility, long-term vision, being gracious with yourself and others, and getting to a place where you can truly enjoy, without guilt, the things you want to enjoy.

SUPPORT THE ECONOMY THROUGH DIETING

Of course, all diet books encourage you in some method that works—if you'll do it. Again, use them as much as you want to. There's a lot of good information out there. And I mean *a lot.*

Actually, one positive thing about the abundance of diet books is that they are good for the economy. I don't have the numbers to support it, but my hunch is that diet books have been a healthy chunk of the U.S. GNP in the last decade. Americans may be getting fatter, but the good news is that our anxiety about weight gain keeps us in the bookstores, picking up the latest, greatest diet plan—and, oh yeah, buying a large mocha latte. Six months later, when our favorite actor has lost thirty pounds on the latest, greatest diet, we'll be back in the bookstore, picking up another diet book and another large latte. It may not make us slim, but at least we're helping the economy stay strong.

There is another benefit—seriously—to all the diet books out there. Every time I read a new diet book, I become highly motivated to focus on my health, even if just for a few months. So in the midst of your Jerusalem Diet, I recommend that you read other diet, nutrition, and exercise books. Why? Because as you accumulate knowledge, you will slowly transition your lifestyle into better eating and more exercise. And in the midst of this, you will be motivated to try some of the diets you are reading about. They may or may not do the trick by themselves, but all of them will help move you along the path of lifestyle transformation. Most of what you incorporate from these diets will improve your life.

Many popular diet plans are great. The problem for me was that I wasn't great at staying 100 percent with them. Most required too much thinking or planning or preparation. And they could do nothing about the problem of easy availability of the "wrong" foods. I could get excited about a diet that had me eating nothing but cucumbers, but after two days, I would drive past an Arby's, and the roast beef with Arby's sauce would call my name. It was soooo easy to pop into the drive-through and get a sandwich, curly fries, and a chocolate shake. Even if I managed to drive past, a Burger King would be on the next block and a KFC on the block after that. Anything I wanted was within a five-minute drive. Why would I want to forsake that kind of variety?

All the diets I have tried have worked…until I didn't want to do them anymore, until I wanted to taste some forbidden food.

Studies suggest that the recidivism rate for diets is about 95 percent.[2] My hunch is that the successful 5 percent are people who wrote the diet plans and who, in essence, get paid to follow them. Maybe the solution is for all of us to write diet books! (But read the opening of this chapter again, and you'll see how well that's working for me.)

Maybe the problem is the word itself: *diet.* Think about it for a moment—what does it connote to you? Dr. Keith-Thomas Ayoob from the American Dietetic Association has suggested that *diet* is no longer a helpful term, because it suggests something temporary—limited to a certain time, a certain trend. There's nothing inherent in the word that contains such parameters, but over time the term has become associated in our culture with failure, with sneaking around, with things that don't last very long, because we all know we can only take so much dieting before we're lining up outside Applebee's for a berry lemon cheesecake. So the word *diet* rings of something we might want to avoid. It suggests that something is over (e.g., your ability to enjoy certain foods) and that, worse, someone has lost (not weight, but a battle).

Perhaps the worst association with the word *diet* is the long list of noes.

No soda. No ice cream. No Snickers. No coffee. No rice. No butter. No cookies. No salt. Going on a diet means you stop enjoying much of what you like about eating. That might hold some adventure for a day or two, but it's tough to make it last.

Diets are reverse psychology in practice. The more you eliminate because of your diet, the more aware you will be of how much you've eliminated. There's nothing like telling yourself, "No carbs for a month!" to make you crave crusty french bread and fettuccine Alfredo. Diets, in this sense, just don't work. We ask for them to be helpful, simple, and dependable, and instead they are antagonizing, complicated, and doomed to failure. They all work—they must, right?—but none of them seem to work for many of us.

Too Many Cooks in the Kitchen

The complexity of the diet guides, systems, and programs available can have a dizzying effect on the national conscience. Here's a game you can play on a lazy Saturday: spend ten minutes in the food and health section at Borders and see how many times you can find experts contradicting each other. This isn't a criticism of real nutritionists and diet-book authors but rather an acknowledgment that the label "expert" gets thrown around with too much ease. If our nation's dieting habits can be thought of as one large kitchen, then we have a problem of too many cooks.

In February 2000 the U.S. Department of Agriculture sponsored a panel of dieting experts to advise Americans how to eat well. They called it the Great Nutrition Debate and packed the panel with some legendary heavy hitters, including the authors of some of the best-selling diet guides of all time: Dr. Robert C. Atkins, Dr. Barry Sears (*The Zone*), Dr. Morrison Bethea (*Sugar Busters!*), as well as other nutritionists and researchers unaffiliated with any popular diet program. The debate lasted three hours, was broadcast on television, and was heavily covered by the media.

The result was a cacophony of advice. One expert encouraged a diet that focused on cutting fatty foods. Another said fat wasn't the problem but carbohydrates were. Another said that plenty of other countries use carbs as a staple, so we needed to reembrace carbs and be concerned about red meats. On and on it went.

Again, I love the free market and love that we are at liberty to test ideas, let them succeed or fail, and then try new ones. But the Great Nutrition Debate is a picture-perfect example of what it can be like to be a health-conscious American today: viewing a panel like that, watching the evidence pile up before you, being bewildered by it all, and leaving you with the sense that you—a nonexpert—are more confused than before, because the experts can't seem to agree on anything except that vegetables are good for you and exercise is important.

THE PROGRESS OF KNOWLEDGE

The debate was just a condensed version of something we've all experienced over our lifetimes. How many of us have become skeptical of any nutrition advice we hear on the news, because we suspect that the advice will flip-flop in a few years? Remember when researchers began to be concerned about the dangers of high cholesterol and its links to heart disease? They told us to stop eating eggs to reduce our cholesterol levels. Researchers kept fiddling with tests and results, and they eventually found that, in moderation, eggs are not life threatening. So all that advice and the creation of new buying habits of American consumers were all for naught.

This seems like flip-flopping to consumers, but in truth, this is how knowledge progresses. When the gurus say, "Lay off proteins," and then later come back screaming, "Increase your protein intake!" and then, "But not animal proteins!" they aren't being contradictory. They are learning. Following developments in nutrition today is like peeping through the window of a scientific laboratory. The scientists are hard at work. Experiments are happening. Instead of reading about the various experiments in the *New England Journal of Medicine,* we're reading best-selling diet books. One experiment is going to improve upon another, and we'll learn more and more over time.

Of course, in my metaphor, it means that we're both the viewers *and* the lab rats. Hmmmm. But that's okay with me. As long as they are not dogmatically telling us to *only* eat foods sold in a particular supermarket or to *only* eat foods prepared a certain way, I'm okay with experimental advice. Diet books should be treated with suspicion, but they should also be seen as

This program is easy, practical, and forgiving, unlike other diets that are strict and difficult for me to follow. What's nice about this program is that I am allowed to eat what my family eats; I don't have to make special meals just for me (unless it is one of my fruits, [vegetables], nuts, seeds, and water days!). The shopping is easy, because my children can eat the same healthy food I am eating.

When I dieted in the past, I felt so hungry that I would end up overeating, then get discouraged and give up the program altogether. With this program, I can accept myself as I am and work toward a manageable weight-loss goal.

I purchased a digital scale and lots of good, healthy food for home and work. I've already started grazing on good foods instead of junk. In the future I plan to invest in a high-powered blender and a juicer.

Thank you again for starting me on the road to health and wellness.

Sylvia

an opportunity to test the latest research that has the potential to improve our lives.

So read and utilize any plan you want, but keep the one-pound-a-week decline as your overall guide, knowing that if you get tired of your new diet, you've still made progress, increased your knowledge, and can continue with the simple Jerusalem Diet plan.

ISN'T THIS A DIET BOOK?

I want to stress that this book is not meant to be the end-all, be-all of diet plans. The Jerusalem Diet is a strategy for living well and enjoying life, not merely getting you to drop weight. In this book I want to give you a plumb line for applying all the ideas you learn about food and health from all reputable sources.

I could no more authoritatively tell you to avoid carbs for a month than I could tell you to learn German; I have no business talking about such things. But I am a pastor, so I can encourage you in life principles. I can help you develop a view of life and health that is simple and doable.

If anyone tells you that the Jerusalem Diet is too easy, blame it on my love of life and simplicity. I like to keep things simple. I don't want to think too hard about what I eat every day. I want to know what's available to me, and I want it to be within reach. I don't want to have to use a special oven or griddle. I don't want to have to shop only at farmers' markets.

This health plan is simple. It takes some discipline, but only a little at a time. It's a slow lifestyle adjustment, not a major overhaul.

Again, read all the diet books and benefit from them. Draw ideas from them. Gain insights. In every diet, nutrition, or exercise book I've read, I've gained at least one essential insight.

Learn about the good fat that comes from oils and the dangers of trans fats. Learn about the benefits of water. Learn about the importance of daily exercise.

Treat diet books like news articles—learn from them. Apply them to your storehouse of knowledge. But stick to the overall plan of the Jerusalem Diet, and you'll have overall long-term success.

CHAPTER 5

Change Your Life...Slowly

The insights that occurred to me that day in Jerusalem have made a slow but permanent impact on my life. In truth, however, I'd been picking up nutrition and exercise tidbits for decades. The way I eat now is different from the way I ate when I was thirty. These changes have occurred over a great deal of time. Nothing happened overnight. Every revolutionary change I made in my eating habits—*No meals after seven o'clock! No carbohydrates at dinner!*—was abandoned within weeks. But the slow, natural, gradual changes I've made have stuck and become an enduring part of my diet.

I know in our fast-and-faster culture there's very little support for the idea, but, really, gradual change is better. Doing things slowly, deliberately, and *for good* is better than doing them quickly and sloppily, only to have to do them all over again.

Relatively speaking, losing your belly fat is no problem. You could go on a crash diet and get it done. Actors gain weight for roles and lose it very quickly, and it's not because they are better people than we are. Think about those actors who give birth to twins and six weeks later are making a movie about the world's skinniest ninja. How is that possible? Well, they employ a staff of experts in weight loss and exercise (not to mention child rearing), and they can spend all day, every day, focused on getting themselves into shape for the next role. In a serious pinch, they also can resort to plastic surgery.

Most of us can't do those things, but we have the capacity to trim our waists. We could eat nothing but cucumbers and broccoli and walk fifteen miles a day, and we'd lose the weight. We'd have to rearrange our entire lives to make it happen, but it would be possible. Regular people do it all the time when they get ready to fit into a wedding dress or go on a beach vacation.

But six months after the wedding and at some point *during* their vacation (if my own vacation habits are any indication), the pounds come right back on. Cucumbers and broccoli work for only so many days in a row. At some point you break down and have a baked potato.

Okay, so how do we get around this problem? How do we begin to embrace gradual change and not worry about fast-track success?

WHY YOU WEIGH WHAT YOU WEIGH

One place to begin is to think more carefully about how you eat and why. Why do you weigh what you weigh? For many people, the first step to health may be in realizing that their weight is not the result of a single factor—their passion for caramels, for instance. Or their genetic makeup. Or their particular culture. Weight is a combination of several elements, including (but not limited to) genes, food environment, eating tendencies, and physical activity.

Your Genes

Your genetic makeup does play a significant role in what you weigh. Studies of adopted children have shown that their weight is determined more by their biological parents than their adoptive parents. If, like me, you come from parents who were heavy, you may feel the diet deck is stacked against you.

But obesity can be a self-fulfilling prophecy. The fact that you come from a line of overweight people does not mean that you are doomed to poor health. You may never have your dream body, but if the goal is overall health and wellness, you can achieve that. The Centers for Disease Control, which performs studies on genomics and obesity, argues that genes are not destiny.[1] You can work with the body you have to improve your health. You can reduce your weight over the total trajectory of your life and are likely to be more healthy and satisfied as a result.

Your Food Environment

Walter Willett, the renowned nutrition researcher, author, and professor at the Harvard School of Public Health, has said that part of the problem facing eaters in America (which is to say, all of us) is that we're surrounded by opportunities to eat.[2] When we stop for gas, we can grab some Corn Nuts and a Sprite. When we go to the grocery store, the checkout line offers a rack of enticing candy bars. The bank has cookies, and most offices offer a bowl of candy. The rise of the coffee culture in the last decade means that many of us have fatty, caffeinated (or decaf) drinks a couple of times a day, perhaps with biscotti or snickerdoodle cookies on the side.

In addition to this, we all have a food culture in our homes that contributes to our overall health or lack thereof. I'll say more about adjusting food practices in your home in the next chapter, but for now let's note that we can do little about the environment we're born into. I opened this book with a celebration of my family's love of food, and I truly did and do love it. But that environment was eventually a problem for my parents' health.

So how do we change a culture? We create a better one. If we want to adjust things in our food environment, we have to be the agents of change.

Your Eating Tendencies

How much weight do you gain while watching the Red Sox–Yankees playoffs on the tube? How much do you eat while waiting for the presidential election results to roll in? If there's a blip in your job or a bump in your marriage, do you sink your face into the food bag?

On the other hand, are you unable to eat for days at a time? During times of stress, do you find yourself nauseated by the thought of food?

What do you eat during your favorite television shows? What do you normally eat after worship services? What's your first food thought of the day? What do you normally munch on between dinner and bedtime?

The last thing I want to do is make you obsess about these things, especially if you're already knee-deep in concern. But if you are not familiar with your food tendencies, it might help to think through an average day or week of eating.

Debt counselors often tell their clients to spend a month writing down every penny they spend, whether it's for a pack of gum at 7-Eleven or a phone bill. That is often the first step to financial freedom, because people's eyes are opened to spending habits that have gone unobserved. Often the shock of learning that Starbucks receives ninety hard-earned bucks a month is motivation enough to limit the latte intake.

Likewise, you might keep a food journal for a week or at least for several days. Document every morsel you eat, without changing your normal routine. Then you will have a record to look over and evaluate. You may be impressed—you may find that the nagging guilt is false guilt and that you aren't doing all that bad. You may find that cutting out midmorning snacks or switching from pastries to eggs for breakfast is the most significant change you need to make. On the other hand, seeing it all before you, line by line, might show you that you're eating far more than you thought you were.

This shouldn't be an exercise in guilt. It should be an exercise in knowledge. Gain insight into what you do and when. "Know thyself."

Your Physical Activity

I'll devote a longer section to exercise later, but for now consider how your daily activity level contributes to your overall body weight and health.

I've written a lot about my family's culture of food, but we also had a solid culture of activity. We lived on a farm with a long list of daily chores. Like many small-town folks, we walked a lot. The Haggard kids played outdoors for hours on end and went inside for dinner only after being called (and called and called). We actually had a dinner bell!

There's no doubt that, as a society, we're less physically active than in the past. Adults and children alike watch an average of four hours of television per day in America, and television viewing is widely considered a leading indicator of obesity.[3]

Consider: Where do you park when you go to the mall? How close do you try to get to the entrance? If you live a half mile or so from any regular destinations—the park, grocery store, post office, church—do you ever walk? Elevators or stairs—which do you choose? In the sum of your life each week, do you find yourself avoiding physical activity, or do you look for places to stretch yourself a bit?

These are some of the elements that account for your weight and health. Notice that you can have an impact on all of them—even the effects of your genetic makeup. You are not glued to where you are. You are not doomed to failure. If you commit to change your life slowly, you can change it permanently and for the better.

ONE DAY, ONE WEEK AT A TIME

As I've mentioned, my mother was dramatically overweight, especially in her later years. When she was at 250 pounds, she would get advice from doctors and various other people. They would say, "Okay, Rachel, we are going to put you on this diet until you are at 200 pounds."

Just from hearing the numbers, she was already defeated. A fifty-pound gap was impossible for her. She just couldn't conceive of ever reaching that goal, and the statement of the obvious—that she was vastly overweight—was enough to convince her that it was a waste of time to even try to diet her way to health.

Sometimes my mother would hear that this pill or that pill would get her down to a normal size, or she'd hear that a particular diet regimen or piece of exercise technology was the guaranteed solution. But those promises were never realized. Mom would buy what they told her to buy, fail, and then get a little more overweight. Next she felt guilty about spending the money…guilty about failing…guilty about weighing too much. She ended up discouraged and would quit. Again and again.

What my mom needed was for someone to tell her, "Rachel, you are at your target weight for this week! Congratulations. You are okay." She needed a simple, doable goal. She needed to be told that she was at her week's target weight and that if she lost just one pound, she'd be on target the next week. She needed realism, and she needed comfort. She needed to be liberated to enjoy her life and have fun improving it a little bit at a time. I'm sad that my ideas on the Jerusalem Diet came after her death.

When I spoke about the Jerusalem Diet at the conference for pastors I mentioned in the introduction, I, of course, emphasized the importance of staying in touch with your health through daily weighing and weekly one pound weight loss. The next year when I spoke at the same conference, a pastor came up to me, carrying a suit.

"This was the suit I wore a year ago," he said, beaming. It was much larger than the one he currently wore. He explained that he had been seriously overweight and had spent years trying and failing at diet plans. "The one-pound-a-week thing made it click for me," he explained. By concentrating on small goals, he was able to address his health in a more natural way. He never mentioned his diet to anyone in his church nor made his program obvious. But he had dropped at least a pound a week and was truly a fraction of his former self.

GRADUAL CHANGE, PERMANENT CHANGE

I am writing this chapter in Dayton, Ohio, where I'm speaking to a national conference of church leaders. My traveling companion on this trip is John Bolin, who serves as an associate pastor with me at New Life Church. While we were out jogging earlier today, we talked about the principle of losing weight slowly, and I told him that our bodies resist rapid weight loss. Often a structural change in our bodies is required to adjust to radical weight changes. So to protect itself, our bodies will fight against quick weight shifts. No doubt, gaining weight is easier than losing weight. But even gaining weight happens slowly for most people.

I've read that many people gain weight at the rate of one pound a year. John and I discovered that we each had gained between one and two pounds a year since graduating from college. We did it slowly and without noticing much. Because of this, even though we want to get back to our college size quickly, our bodies will fight that process if we try to make it happen too rapidly. Why? We have adjusted, over years, to our new weight.

But consider: on the Jerusalem Diet, you can lose fifty-two pounds in a year! That still might be too fast. In a special weight-loss issue of *Men's Health* in 2005, there was a series of testimonies from men who successfully lost significant weight and kept it off for more than a year. The most compelling testimony was from Mark Davis, who once weighed 368 pounds but dropped to 200 pounds. His story is both amazing and instructive:

Bay Area resident Mark Davis shrank from 235 pounds to 175 in just 12 weeks using a crash diet, then rebounded all the way up to 368 pounds. After an embarrassing episode on a theme-park ride (the restraining bar wouldn't fit over him), he vowed to lose the weight for good. He started with an exercise bike, working up from 2 minutes a day at the lowest intensity to 30 minutes at the highest. Then he took up weight training. Four years later, he was down to 200 pounds. "I lost the weight slowly," Davis says. "That's the biggest mistake people make—they think it's a race. I lost eight-tenths of a pound each week for 4 years."[4]

Aha! Mark's success came gradually over time and involved both exercise and diet.

Slow, steady transition. This is why the Jerusalem Diet is an overall plan for gradual weight, diet, and exercise adjustment utilizing a steady accumulation of information from many popular diet, exercise, and nutrition programs.

I'll never forget when my wife and I read Dr. Rex Russell's book, *What the Bible Says About Healthy Living*. It changed our way of evaluating food. Russell basically says that the closer food is to its original creation, the better it is for you. Three big ideas are the basis of the book:

1. *Eat the foods God created for you.* Russell says that the best medicine for good health is good food. He argues that the top ten reasons for hospitalization in the United States (obesity, diabetes, hemorrhoids and varicose veins, heart attacks, diverticulosis and diverticulitis, cancer, peptic ulcer, hiatal hernia, appendicitis, and gallstones) can all be positively affected by an improved diet. It doesn't happen overnight. We can't mistreat our bodies for years, get sick, and then think that we can eat better for a few months and be well. We need to start slowly improving our lives now by eating good food.

2. *Don't alter God's design.* Russell says that life doesn't have to be as random as many think. We can cooperate with God's plan, walk in obedience, and receive the benefits, or we can go our own way and receive some of the consequences. The obvious application to nutrition is whether or not we eat food close to the way nature provides

it. If we want to endlessly process and refine food, we may learn to our detriment that there are negative consequences. Whole-grain wheat bread versus superprocessed white bread. An apple versus cotton candy. Broadly, these are some of our choices.

3. *Don't let any food or drink become your god.* Russell balances all of our lives by saying that even though food is the best medicine, no food can be good medicine. He discusses the biblical exhortations to fast—to go without food for a few days and let our systems rest and recover from constant use.[5] I'm not a proponent of extended fasts unless you think you might be another Jesus or Moses, but a good one-to-three-day fast a few times a year can do wonderful things for our bodies and our hearts.

The Jerusalem Diet is not about fasting, so I'll not comment on it much. But I do believe that everyone would benefit from taking a few days off to pray and fast in a quiet place. It provides great spiritual and physical benefits. But let me emphasize: three days is probably enough. Then eat and return to your routine. If you want to fast again, wait a month or two.

Okay, now back to the main point. Slow weight adjustment is the key, and this comes from a gradual shift in lifestyle. You may be like me, in that to make a significant lifestyle change, several radical attempts at alterations may be required before you finally are able to be consistently careful about what you eat and how you exercise. For example, go on Atkins for a month to learn about simple and complex carbohydrates and protein and their effects on your body. A month on Atkins will permanently inform you about some foods and will therefore impact your eating habits in the future. Once you're off Atkins, you still will have shifted toward better food. Real change requires a lifestyle alteration, which takes time.

The National Weight Control Registry (NWCR) from the University of Pittsburgh documents people who have lost weight and maintained their new, lower weight. The program searches for people who have lost at least thirty pounds and kept it off for one year or longer. They have four thousand people in their registry who have dropped pounds and kept them off. Remarkably, while thirty pounds was the threshold to be included in the study, their first report was made up of people who had lost an average of more than sixty pounds! Even more remarkable, nearly half of the participants reported that keeping the weight off was much easier than initially losing the weight.[6]

Did you catch that? Losing the weight was *harder* than keeping it off. This is very different from what many of the best-selling diet guides lead us to believe in their "Six Weeks to Trim Up!" marketing tactics. The hurdle to begin a diet and start having success can be tough, but the people in the NWCR reported that once they leaped that hurdle, they felt their lives were restored. All reported elevated self-confidence, mood, and overall health. They relearned the basic skills of eating and exercise. They approached life differently and cooking and grocery shopping differently. A paradigm shift truly occurred.

What did these people have in common? Over an extended period of time, they began to eat healthier foods and exercise more. They burned more calories than they took in. They still ate the high-fat foods they loved, but eventually they learned to enjoy them in moderation.

That was it. There was no other common factor. They lost their weight in different ways with different plans. No sudden-loss, crash diets. No quick fixes. No "eat what you want, don't exercise, but just take our pill" plans or "As Seen on TV" exercise systems. Just gradual change. Continual change. Permanent change.

INTERNAL AND EXTERNAL CONTROL

Let me make one more important point about incorporating change. In order to do it, we need both internal and external control.

Most often, married people are healthier than unmarried people. They live longer, eat better, exercise more often, have more active social lives, and have fewer accidents. Why? Because they watch out for each other.

The other night I was watching television, and I asked Gayle if she would bring me a bowl of ice cream. She answered, "Do you want me to help you live a longer life?"

A year ago I walked out of the gym and stopped my healthy eating habits. I don't know if I was burned out or just needed a break. After twelve months I had gained thirty-five pounds, was tired, and felt lousy. (This is not a good trend when you teach students outdoor skills!) I felt drained spiritually, too. I looked in the mirror and knew something had to change.

I have been following the Jerusalem Diet along with the Body-for-Life lifestyle. I have lost fifteen pounds and need to shed fifteen more to reach my ideal weight.

I love the simplicity and gradual loss of pounds. The Fat Days are great. I already had a high-powered blender, but I hadn't done tomatoes in it. That's a great idea, and it only takes minutes during a hurried morning. I don't feel sluggish at all anymore.

Because of adopting healthier eating habits and adding exercise to my day, I have more energy and sleep better at night. I love that I can use the Jerusalem Diet as a stand-alone guide or adapt it to be used with other programs.

Another great thing about this diet is how easy it is to share with others. It only takes five minutes to explain the whole plan. People can't believe it is that simple. But it is!

Ruth-Ann

Grrrr. I hate it when she says things like that. I gave in to the urge: "Start that tomorrow. I want ice cream!"

This is why married people live longer. We gripe at each other. We encourage each other. We watch out for each other. Every husband knows the sound of his wife's encouragement to eat salad instead of fried shrimp. Every mom knows the concern of seeing her family slide toward unhealthy habits and their consequences.

Families also provide external constraints. A meal prepared at home is more likely to be good for you than the bag of burgers and onion rings purchased at a fast-food restaurant. Single people living alone can arrange the same type of accountability with friends or extended family members.

We all need to develop internal constraints as well. It's natural to eat more than we should, and processed food is inexpensive, easily available, and tasty. As a result, we must be intentional about our diets and our health.

Food manufacturers don't profit when we don't eat. There is no economic incentive for them to encourage us to eat smaller portions. So the decision has to come from us. We have to take responsibility for what we eat.

But we need external and internal motivation. When I travel, I occasionally pick up a copy of *Men's Health* or *Men's Fitness*. I don't typically read these magazines, but glancing at them once in a while provides motivation for me.

Walking through the mall and looking at people also provides motivation for me. The overweight ones motivate me to never look the way they do. The fit ones motivate me to watch what I eat and to be physically active.

I have exercise equipment at home. But when I get tired of working out there, I use my membership at 24-Hour Fitness to gain motivation. How? When I go to the club, I see men and women who look great! Seeing both those who are younger and those who are older than I am keeping their bodies healthy and strong motivates me.

Oddly, a visit to the health-food store does not give me that same motivation. Why is it that some of the most pale and frail-looking people I've ever seen are the ones who shop at health-food stores? Maybe they have been sick and are trying to save their lives, or maybe they have overindulged in the health-food culture and are suffering from it. They might actually be healthier by having a hamburger and going to 24-Hour Fitness instead.

John Bolin and I got some motivation yesterday when we arrived at our hotel. The man who checked us in was so overweight he couldn't bend over. He had to spread his legs as far apart as possible and lean sideways in order to reach down. John and I went running that day, ate only good food, and drank lots of water. We didn't talk about it; we were just motivated to live better lives. It made me wish the Jerusalem Diet book was already published so the man at the hotel desk could hear that small, doable goals could save his life. I guarantee that he hates his weight and his appearance. He's probably tried all kinds of programs, but the road they offered was too long. He needs this plan. He needs to know he can lose one pound and start his journey from there.

One pound a week. That's all it takes—slow, steady, and doable.

CHAPTER 6

Change Your Home's Culture

L ast summer a friend of mine, Daniel Grothe, and I were running partners. Every day or two we would pound the pavement for a while, then go back to my house and throw several oranges into the blender. As we stood in the kitchen with our clothes still wet and drops of sweat falling from our foreheads, we would gulp down big glasses of living nutrients. Ahhhh. We could feel nutrition going straight to our cells.

Sometimes we'd blend strawberries and apples and drink the mix. We felt so alive—running in the crisp Colorado air, wearing ourselves out, then recuperating with a genuinely pure fruit or vegetable drink. We'd worked our hearts and muscles hard, then rewarded them with nutrients. Our bodies seemed to rejoice at the pure food pouring into our systems.

I love our blender! There's nothing quite like taking seedless grapes and making a fresh glass of authentic grape juice. It tastes better than anything I've found in the store, and it's loaded with nutrients. And since the machine isn't just a juicer but a high-powered mixer, I keep the pulp, the fiber—the whole fruit—and drink it all.

I also enjoy strawberries and apples with a banana. Or, on some mornings, I take a whole cucumber, wash it off, and put it into my juicer rather than the more powerful blender. I don't want to eat the skin of the cucumber, but I do want the liquid and nutrients from the cucumber. After juicing a whole cucumber, I drink it down. It tastes like I'm drinking my freshly cut yard! I feel so alive I could moo!

Juicing a cucumber may make you wonder if you are a cow, but you'll know you are pouring a great combination of vitamins and minerals into your system. Multivitamins are good, and I take them every day, but even the best of them don't do what real, whole fruits and vegetables can do.

Later in this book you'll see a section with more information on drinking fruits and vegetables. So why am I introducing the topic now? Because I want you to get the whole picture of our lives at home. What's made scenes like the previous one possible is that over the years Gayle and I have transitioned our home culture so the family enjoys real food. We've created a culture of health in our home.

We're a juicer family. We're a blender family. We have concentrated juices in the fridge as well, but most often, rather than grabbing a prepackaged juice, I reach for whatever is on the counter—carrots, kiwis, apples—and either eat them as a snack or throw them into the blender.

Our kids watch my wife and me do this, and consequently, they do it too. When they exercise or play hard, they often mix fruits or vegetables in the blender or juicer and drink real food as a refreshment afterward.

Not long ago I walked into the kitchen on a Saturday afternoon and saw our twelve-year-old son, Elliott, at the table with several of his friends. Elliott had put our blender on the counter and was showing his buddies what it could do.

"Check this out!" he said, pushing a series of apples, bananas, strawberries, and then some oranges into the machine. *Whirrrrrrrr!* "Now watch this!" he yelled, adding tangerines and anything else within reach. *Whirrrrrrrr!* After he'd packed the blender to his friends' delight and turned the liquid inside into a whole range of bright colors, he poured everyone a big glass.

"Mmmm, that's awesome!" they all agreed.

I got a thrill out of watching them, because I could remember being

Elliott's age and showing my buddies all the great sugary goodies Mom had baked over the weekend and then stuffing our faces with cookies, doughnuts, and homemade fudge. But here Elliott was (unwittingly, of course) showing his buddies just how much fun it can be to have a healthy snack.

No doubt, sometimes a cupcake is delightful—especially a Hostess cupcake with that great creamy, sugary center. But the people in my home find themselves desiring these less and less.

CHANGE YOUR CULTURE...SLOWLY

The Haggard health culture didn't happen overnight, and that's the point of this chapter. If you try to change your life, diet, and exercise routine in a day because you saw a video or read a book, you will likely fail. Instead, watch the video and read the book, but do it within an overall plan like the Jerusalem Diet. Gradually transition your life. Take your time and create a healthy lifestyle that makes sense for you and your family.

I'm not saying you should be passive. I am saying that if you try to lose weight too fast, your body won't adjust quickly enough, and you'll most likely lose the battle against fat. If you try to change your home overnight, your kids will end up laughing at you, remembering the health-food craze Mom went through when she had disgusting food all around the house.

Instead, change slowly. Lose one pound a week. Find real, good food you like and keep it around. Find exercise habits that work for you. Find a way of life that makes sense and promotes health and good humor around your home.

Gayle has done a great job of changing the culture of our home. Where the kitchen used to be stocked with M&M's, baked beans, macaroni and cheese, and sugary cereals, now there are bowls of grapes, carrot sticks, yogurt, and cheese. A huge pile of fruit sits on the kitchen counter, and the kids grab from it all day long.

Don't get me wrong. We are Jerusalem Diet people, which means we haven't ditched junk or comfort foods entirely. On the Fourth of July, we had hamburgers, hot dogs, baked beans, potato salad, chips and salsa, guacamole, fruit salads, and strawberry shortcake, along with the usual range of drinks. The next day I was two pounds over my target, so I ate fruits, vegetables, nuts, and seeds. For exercise, I ran for thirty minutes on the treadmill and swam in the pool for thirty minutes. Consequently, the next morning I was one pound under my target weight! I don't think anyone ever noticed.

Yeah, I still love Jelly Bellies and Mountain Dew—but the culture of our lives is changing.

FLEXIBILITY AND FAT DAYS

I'm in Vail, Colorado, now as I'm writing. Gayle and I are taking a couple of days to get away together and work on this book. (Women, be sure to check out Gayle's fantastic chapter, if you haven't already!) Because there is no scale in my hotel room, I have to guess at my weight. But I've done this long enough that I can tell with fair accuracy if I'm overweight or not.

Yesterday I was underweight. I could have eaten whatever I wanted. But after Gayle and I woke up, we ordered room service late in the morning—two fruit plates with yogurt. Through the balance of the morning and into late afternoon, I grazed on that fruit plate.

Then, during the evening news, I had a normal meal of salad, beef, a baked potato, and some vegetables. At 8:30 we decided to catch the late showing of *Cinderella Man*. When we got to the theater, we each ordered a small popcorn (we know, we know, for only twenty-five cents more, you can get twice as much!) and a small drink (I had Cherry Coke, and Gayle got a Classic Coke). Yes, there are terrible things in theater popcorn and in soda. But we bought small quantities of these two items and were perfectly happy. We didn't talk about it or have to discipline ourselves because of some quota for the day. Instead, we did it naturally because it's our family culture. If this had happened on a Fat Day, I would have ordered a bottle of water and thought during the movie, *Man! Why did I have those nachos and a doughnut yesterday!*

We commonly talk about whether one of us is having a Fat Day. A Fat Day is, as you now know, a code term for being a pound or two above where we are supposed to be that day. So if one of us is having a Fat Day, that person is limited to fruits, vegetables, nuts, seeds, and water to drink. But even when we're not having a Fat Day, we are increasingly likely to eat better food, because we're increasingly aware of an easy method to maintain our ideal weight without being health extremists. So if you walked into our house today, you'd find a great balance of fun food—most of it healthy, some of it decadent.

TOTAL LIFE AND BODY HEALTH

The establishment of the culture of health in our home actually began when I was still in college. I attended a Christian university that taught that our bodies are a gift from God for us to use to serve others. They said that in order for us to fulfill God's plan for our lives, our bodies had to be well maintained.

I think they were right. For our lives to be complete, we need to maintain our bodies and keep them healthy. We also need to develop a healthy spiritual life, and we need to be mentally strong. My university required that we exercise, attend chapel and Sunday church services off campus, and go to class diligently. Since Gayle and I met in college in the midst of this atmosphere, we were both persuaded of the importance of physical, spiritual, and mental health.

As newlyweds, we would often jog together as well as pray together. When the children came along, they saw us exercising, participating in our local church, and reading and discussing books at home. As the years have passed, we've continued with this practice of physical, spiritual, and mental growth. We regularly exercise, we believe in God and the principles of the Bible, and we love to read and discuss ideas.

In our home we don't watch television during June, July, and August. We're outside more and involved in more physical activities. Don't get me wrong—we aren't all health all the time. For Father's Day this year, the family bought me a portable firepit so we can have open fires in our backyard during the evenings without the fire department being called. So we've eaten more roasted marshmallows than normal. But, culturally speaking, the Haggards are outdoorsy, active folks.

Because that's our culture, we've kept up with the newest nutrition, diet, and exercise information as it's become available. Most recently we enjoyed *The Maker's Diet* by Jordan Rubin. Jordan is a personal friend, and we've done everything we can to encourage people in our sphere of influence to read and apply the principles in *The Maker's Diet*. The products that Jordan has developed are excellent too, and Gayle and I take some of them regularly. In our opinion, this is the best set of materials available to date.

Before *The Maker's Diet*, we enjoyed what Dr. Atkins taught us. We also enjoyed *The South Beach Diet, Eat Right 4 Your Type,* Dr. Kenneth Cooper's materials on aerobics and preventive health, and many others. They are all helpful and contribute to our overall knowledge of health and nutrition.

Because these books and ideas are a part of the culture of the Haggard home, our kids have grown up hearing health discussions—overprocessed (dead) versus real food, water versus soda, exercise versus laziness, and all the variations therein. The kids assimilate these ideas on nutrition and exercise and have varieties of ideas floating around in their brains, so they know how to evaluate new information as they hear it.

It's not unusual to see Christy, our twenty-three-year-old daughter, running three to five miles a day. Often she can be seen munching on celery and carrot sticks, though she's not dogmatic about it. She and her four brothers have a healthy view of body, mind, and spirit. They are good students, they enjoy their local church, they lead honorable lives in the community, and they are physically fit.

Fitness Culture

Fitness is a culture. It's a lifestyle. It's not something you reprogram over the course of six weeks. It's the gradual creation of a way of life.

Earlier I wrote about all our associations with the word *diet*—limitations, short-term projects, a long list of noes, and so forth. You might find it interesting that the word *diet* comes from the Greek word *diaita,* which has to do with a *way of life*—a lifestyle, a way of being. In our contemporary parlance, *diet* pertains only to what we eat, but it would be helpful if we could recover some of the original meaning and understand how much diet has to do with a total lifestyle.

I've not said much about spirituality in this book, because that is not my focus for this project. I've written other materials on spirituality that you can pick up if you wish. But I do want to impress upon you the importance of modeling healthy ideas to help those around you to be happy and successful.

As I've said, I am a leader of a church. I believe it's important for me and the others who serve from the platform of our church to be relatively fit and to look like normal people—not inappropriately dressed or overly groomed. On the other hand, we shouldn't be overweight, out of shape, or sloppy. Since I serve as the senior pastor, I am intentional about what is portrayed on our platform. I ask that the men and women on the platform live their lives—not just their spiritual lives but their whole lives—in a way that models helpful ideas for those who see and listen to us week after week.

Because of this, we have a great-looking team. Now, I cringe a little as I write this, because I fear that you are thinking of the overly made-up, performance types who sometimes are on religious television programs. Nope, I'm not describing the self-absorbed; I'm describing the opposite. I'm talking about healthy people who are not self-consumed or self-conscious. I'm talking about people who don't primp constantly but are fit because they practice total health.

I love having these people around me, and I love letting them model well-lived lives for the people in our church.

DIET MATTERS

Let me encourage you a little bit on changing the culture of your home. I want you to have a great time on this diet, and obviously I have fun kidding around with these ideas, but for a moment I want to say something about the great benefits of orienting the culture of your home toward health.

Dr. Walter Willett at the Harvard School of Public Health has said that a healthy diet alone—that is, just being careful about nutrition—can result in a longer, more productive life. His studies have suggested that 82 percent of heart attacks, 70 percent of strokes, 90 percent of Type II diabetes, and more than 70 percent of colon cancers can be totally prevented with a healthy diet. Stop and read that sentence again. Don't skim this! Think about it. Dr. Willett made the point that while we put lots of money and energy toward promoting drugs to fight heart disease, the best drugs reduce the chance of a heart attack by only 20–30 percent. In other words, the best drugs are less than half as effective as good nutrition.[1]

Another famous nutritionist, Dr. Ancel Keys from the University of Minnesota—the doctor famous for inventing K rations for American soldiers during World War II—showed how much a healthy cultural environment can contribute to a long, healthy life. (Keys lived until he was nearly 101, so we can be pretty sure he knew what he was talking about!) Keys is the one who told us about the dangers of certain fats and cholesterol, and he's also the one who began to prove that our body type and genetic makeup don't doom us to poor health.

I am forty-six years old. Twenty-three years ago I was a healthy, strong, in-shape young man—then I walked off the farm and into an office. The weight crept up slowly enough for me to deny I had a problem for ten years. As with so many families I know, I grew heavier, and my wife, children, and grandchildren remained wonderfully fit.

I am now in my thirteenth week of the Jerusalem Diet, although today is a "fruits, vegetables, nuttin' sweet" day (I know what it's supposed to say!). I have tried many other things through the years, and what makes this different (for me, anyway) is that

- it is based on acceptance instead of condemnation and guilt;
- it is simple, without a lot of formulas, theories, counters, study, and difficult grocery lists to lug around;
- it's not hard to do and is based on achievable goals.

What gets measured gets managed. I simply put in each week's new target weight on my Palm Pilot and weigh every day (that was a major lifestyle change in itself). I am now 26 percent of my way toward my final target.

It is incredible how out of touch I was with my own body. Now, before I go to bed, I can tell whether or not the next day will be a Fat Day. It is so good to know my body.

I actually enjoy walking now. My feet don't hurt, and I think everything, including my truck seats, will last longer. I also really appreciate not having to burden others with particulars when a meal is offered. In the past I just went off whatever diet I was on at that point, because I never would insult someone who was offering me food. Now I know I can occasionally drive a little left of center, as long as I keep my eye on the hill and don't go too far over.

Carl

Some people have genuine genetic problems, but I'd wager that they are far, far outnumbered by those who just *claim* to have genetic problems. Too many people who struggle with their weight have had someone tell them that they have a genetic predisposition toward obesity and that they will always be fat. Again, I know that there are some cases like this, but most who believe this are using these comments as a crutch.

The bottom line: there is nothing in us that we didn't eat. For the vast majority of us, if we're fat, it's because we ate too much, ate the wrong things, and moved too little. If it's in us, we ate it. If it stayed in us, we didn't move enough between feedings to get rid of it.

We are responsible for our bodies. We can't blame others—such as our parents—our genetics, or our environment. Even though these are factors, we have to take responsibility for who we are, how we eat and exercise, and how we live.

Dr. Keys demonstrated this idea. In one of his studies, he looked at fourteen groups from different regions of Europe and Asia. Those in countries with healthier environments—where more low-fat, natural foods are a common part of the diet—had lower rates of heart disease. But when those people migrated to a place like the United States and took on a higher-fat diet and exercised less, their rates of heart disease rose to match those in their new home country.

This information doesn't seem surprising to us now, but it tells us a lot about how much lifestyle contributes to overall health. Fitness is a culture, and so is unfitness.[2]

START CHANGING YOUR CULTURE NOW

An existing culture is hard to fix. However, a culture can slowly evolve—or a new culture can be created. No matter what state your life or home is in, you can create something better from this day forward.

Relax. Accept yourself. Start where you are. Love the body God gave you, and start taking responsibility for it. Don't launch into a program that will force you to think about every bite you eat, every step you take, and everything you wear. Use your body for God's purpose for your life. Don't live your life for your body.

In our church and in our home we try to reflect the importance of a healthy body so that we can live to our full potential. I'm forty-nine years old. I will never be on the cover of a fitness magazine. I will never be that perfectly molded guy at 24-Hour Fitness who exercises three hours a day. But at the same time, I am fit. I'm at or near my ideal weight. I'm able to have a great time with my family and friends. My mind is strong (depending on whom you ask!), and I am enjoying a dynamic spiritual life. It's a well-balanced life.

You were made for this kind of life too. Enjoy!

CHAPTER 7

Change Your Life's Trajectory

When I walk into restaurants, I look around to see what people are eating. Sometimes there is a direct correlation between people's size and what they choose to eat. Some overweight people are overweight for obvious reasons. As they sit at dinner, drinking soft drink after soft drink to wash down chicken-fried steak and buttery mashed potatoes, their size is easy to explain.

They are eating themselves fat.

For that group of people, the source of their size is clear. But then there's the other, more mysterious group. Sometimes overweight people seem to be doing their best to stick to the latest health-food recommendations—avoiding cheeseburgers and fish 'n' chips in favor of salad, cottage cheese, and water. Yet they remain fat. Most frustrating of all, the skinny people around them seem to eat whatever they want and not gain a pound. Why is that so?

It's the question that plagues many dieters: why can some people eat anything they want and not gain weight, while others get fat on cottage cheese and salad?

The default explanation—you may be already thinking it—is biochemistry. *That's me!* some of you are thinking. *I have bad genes! My body makes any food into fat!* It's a common notion that some people are predisposed to gain weight because of genetics and a sluggish metabolism.

By and large, that's a misconception. As I explained earlier, genetics is just one explanation for why you weigh what you weigh, and it's probably not the best explanation. For most overweight people, biochemistry is not enough of an answer for their weight problem. Even if you come from a gene pool of overweight people, you do not have to be victimized by your genes. And if your metabolism works slowly, you can do things to speed it up, such as exercise.

Be sure you get those two ideas. One: your genes are probably not what make you fat. Two: you can stimulate your metabolism through exercise.

Consider this: scientists have never discovered the gene or genetic makeup that predetermines obesity. While we know that genes play a role in the development of obesity, Dr. Claude Bouchard, an obesity geneticist, has argued that their role is modest at best.[1] Instead, current research suggests that environmental factors play a more determining role in obesity. Your environment creates mentalities and habits that are powerful forces in shaping the direction of your life (and in shaping your body).

We probably can't do much about the environment we came from, but we can do a lot, starting today, about our current environment.

In the last two chapters I encouraged you to slowly change your life and the culture of your home. Now I want to address your responsibility to adjust your approach to eating and exercising. I want to tell you how to be a person of fitness rather than a person of fatness. In other words, if cottage cheese and carrot sticks make you fat, I want to tell you how to change the course of your life so exercise is a joy, not a drudge. I want you on the road toward health, fitness, and happiness rather than sickness, immobility, and depression.

Read on. You're about to learn the central lesson of the Jerusalem Diet.

A Trajectory Toward Being Fit or Fat

A *trajectory* is a powerful force. Once begun, a trajectory can be hard to change. Most trial lawyers will tell you that they can sense early on what the verdict of a case will be, which is why so much care is put into the selection of a jury and opening statements. Financial planners understand this notion too; they won't guide you in dramatic, overnight changes, but they will tell you how to begin to make different choices so that every month can be a little better than the one before. After years of "little better months," you will have created a trajectory toward prosperity.

The reason diets so often fail is that they don't change the trajectory of our eating and exercise habits. They give us great advice that we're able to follow for a little while, but we often don't allow them enough time to redirect our behavior. Our lives are busy, so the quick fix and immediate results offered by some diets are appealing in our harried existence, and we give them a try. But when we regress, we end up disappointed and fat.

A friend of mine recently mentioned the Jerusalem Diet to a nutritionist. The nutritionist couldn't believe what we were recommending—one-day adjustments in the context of gradual life change while not being legalistic about eating decadent foods. "That's crazy!" he said. "How can it be good to do something for only one day? You can't eat one way for one day and then another way the next day." His response was typical. He didn't understand human nature. He obviously didn't think about it, but he was actually saying, "You've either got to be healthy or unhealthy." That nutritionist is going to have a hard time getting anyone to maintain a long-term eating and exercising plan. He's not being realistic about the way people's lives really and permanently change.

Government officials know the importance of establishing a positive trajectory in a person's life. On June 30, 2003, *Food and Drink Weekly* reported on a bill introduced by Democratic Representative Dennis Cardoza and Republican Congressman Adam Putnam trying to encourage school children to eat more fruits and vegetables. In their proposal, Cardoza and Putnam said that America's health depends upon children eating more fruits and vegetables.

Think of this. Leaders in our government know that the future health of the nation is dependent upon improved nutrition, namely, additional fruits and vegetables in our diets. *Food and Drink Weekly* reported, "The bill also would provide small grants for schools to create vegetable gardens to show kids where healthy food comes from." The report continued, "The legislators hope that getting kids to dump fatty or sugar-laden foods in favor of fresh fruits and vegetables could help reverse the national obesity epidemic. Increased childhood obesity is blamed on bad eating habits and a lack of childhood exercise."[2]

The way I see it, if you eat fast-food burgers three days in a row but on the fourth day you stick to fruits, vegetables, nuts, seeds, and water, then at least you've given your body one day of assistance and strength. It's better for you to have a one-day adjustment than never to make good eating decisions. And the more you make one-day adjustments, the more you'll shift your life away from foods that actually work against your body and toward better foods. As you begin the occasional one-day adjustment on your Fat Days, you will put yourself on a trajectory toward fitness.

The Jerusalem Diet is a trajectory-changing diet. It's not about a temporary shift in nutrition or exercise habits. It's not about a sudden break from all the foods you love and the laziness you've carefully and joyfully cultivated throughout your life. The reason I want you to be free to enjoy Baskin-Robbins and lay around for a day is that I'm not interested in sudden and obvious but ultimately temporary adjustments. I'm interested in slow, gradual, permanent change. I'm interested in starting a trend toward health. I'm interested in changing the trajectory of your life.

It's About Choices

Your genes are your genes, your past is your past, and your habits are your habits. But what goes inside your body is up to you.

The reason you can walk into a restaurant and see an overweight person carefully eating cottage cheese and a fit person eating a banana split is because one has consistently made better decisions than the other. One has established a trend toward health; the other has established a trend toward being overweight.

More than likely, the overweight person has the same rate of metabolism as the fit person. However, because of exercise, the fit person has greater muscle mass, and muscle is live, vital tissue that's always consuming energy—burning calories.

Write this on a piece of paper and stick it to your bathroom mirror or car windshield: "There is nothing inside me that I didn't eat." Cause a shift in your paradigm for weight loss. What you do every day—how much you move—is the bulk of the problem and also the majority of the solution.

When we were younger, we could eat all we wanted, and it would hardly affect our weight. Our metabolism was kicking, because we were moving more and building and stimulating muscle. Later in life we slowed down, our muscle mass declined, we needed less energy but—oops—did not lower our intake of food accordingly. If we're overweight, it's because we made ourselves that way.

As I've said before, I'm not a doctor, a chemist, or a nutritionist, nor am I a well-disciplined man. But I am a pastor who watches thousands of people live their lives. I have devoted my life to learning what makes lives better and what causes lives to go awry. I have a clue about why cottage cheese makes some people fat and pizza doesn't cause others to get fat.

Again, the answer is that one group has a trajectory toward fitness; the other doesn't.

Move Your Body—Move Your Metabolism, Too

I know that because of authentic physical limitations, it's more difficult for some people to get fit than others. But regardless of what or who is to blame, if we don't do our best to take responsibility for ourselves and improve ourselves, no one else will. I decided long ago to take what I was given (my genetics, my heritage, my background) and make the best from it to serve others in life. There are plenty of negatives in my genes and my family history that I could focus on. But I've chosen to minimize those negatives and focus on the good and on my potential to change things.

As a result of believing that I should take responsibility for myself and of observing thousands of people up close by virtue of my occupation, I don't believe most people are victims of their metabolism. Actually, regardless of our age, metabolism can be an ally in weight control.

When you and I were kids, we *moved*. We ran, jumped, twirled, twisted, played sports, and fidgeted while sitting in a chair. We didn't stop. We continued to move a lot during our teenage years, which is why most of us didn't start to gain excessive weight until our college years or shortly thereafter.

Many people get married right after college and then blame their additional weight on being married and finally eating good cooking. But the more obvious answer is that they're not moving as much. People start to add fat easily when they aren't moving as much, and with less muscle mass requiring fuel, the body burns fewer calories. They are less fit, and, as a result, their food turns to fat.

A Midchapter Q and A

"Ted, can people improve their metabolism?"

"Yes. More accurately, they can improve the effectiveness of their metabolism."

"How?"

"By exercising and increasing the amount of muscle they have."

"Does food affect everyone the same way?"

"No. Healthy people digest and use food better than fat people."

"Well, how can I ensure that food affects me in the best possible way? How can I ensure that eating cottage cheese and salad will actually make a difference for me?"

"By increasing the rate at which your body burns calories—exercise! By being fit. Move. Build muscle. Start a trend toward health. By making your life trajectory one of overall fitness. Pay close attention to this: If you are fit, food doesn't have the same potential to make you fat. If you are fat, you can diet all you like, but you will probably get fatter no matter what you eat."

"In your opinion, what makes people more healthy—the health-food store or the gym?"

"The gym, because healthy people tend to exercise and eat right. They aren't necessarily all-organic-all-the-time people. They aren't trying to fix all their weight issues at once with low-carb or whole-grain solutions. They are achieving a balance between moving their bodies and eating well. They are on a trajectory toward health."

∞∞∞

If your goal is to lose weight in three weeks to fit into a dress or swimsuit, you can do it. But you're doomed to have short-term success. It'd be much better to grab a calendar and a scale and start the Jerusalem Diet. Have slow, gradual, and permanent change. Have the flexibility to mess up and enjoy sweets. Maintain the long view. Work toward being fit—for good. And while doing this, eat some Popeye's chicken and biscuits.

How Much Body Is Okay?

You should carry only as much fat as good fitness allows. In other words, work on getting your body-fat percentage to a level where you are on a trajectory toward fitness rather than fatness. My experience has been that men do well to have between 15 and 18 percent body fat and women should have between 22 and 25 percent.

Once you reach your ideal weight on the Jerusalem Diet, add resistance training in order to build muscle (that stimulates metabolism), and give yourself more freedom. I'll mention this again later, but let me give you an easy way to begin toning your body.

On your plan you will start at your current weight and then mark on a calendar the number of pounds and weeks it will take for you to reach your ideal weight. If you want to tone up, my advice is to wait until you are about two-thirds of the way toward your goal, then start doing sit-ups (crunches), push-ups, and squats every morning. On the first day, do one of each. On the second, do two. On the third, do three. (See what I mean about slow, steady progress? This is great stuff!) Increase the number you do by one every day until, say, you reach your age.

Let me say a word of caution about squats. If you are quite heavy or out of shape, this exercise may strain your knees too much, so you should avoid them. And you should never dip below ninety degrees in your knee bend; your knee is unstable beyond that point.

These exercises do not count in your hour of exercise for your Fat Days. Instead, they are basic strength-and-movement exercises that won't take long but will help you tone and build muscle. Muscle burns energy. When building muscle and increasing strength, you'll look better, feel stronger, stand and walk with more confidence, and be motivated to eat better.

And guess what else toned muscles do? They make your metabolism work for you. Remember, the primary control mechanism for obesity is not genetics or any particular diet plan; it's metabolism—the rate at which your body burns the calories needed to keep you going. Dieting alone is useful for losing fat temporarily, but it doesn't cure the tendency to easily become fat. To lose the tendency to become fat, you must be fit.

FROM FAT TO FIT

You can become fit. You can start where you are and make gradual changes that improve your life. You may never have the perfect body you want, but that's okay. If you improve your fitness, you'll be healthier and happier. And your idea of the perfect body will become more reasonable.

Later in this book you'll read a chapter entitled "Move Your Body However You Can." But because overall fitness—that is, having a trajectory toward health—is so dependent upon exercise, I want to go over the central concepts here. I do not advocate one strict, regimented exercise routine, but I do encourage you to move your body more and develop a lifestyle and culture of exercise.

I tell people who are horrified at the thought of exercise to do whatever they can to move. One lady told me that all she could do was throw her legs over the edge of her bed and bounce them for a little while. Whatever! It's better to do that than lie motionless in bed.

On Fat Days on the Jerusalem Diet, exercise for one hour. The point of that exercise is not just to burn calories but to introduce fitness to your lifestyle. It's to encourage you to get into the flow of aerobic exercise and resistance training however you can. If you vigorously exercise, you will burn more calories after exercising than while you were exercising. And once you are fit, you'll burn calories while you sleep. It's incredible.

Rather than saying, "Go to the gym, buy a membership, hire a trainer, and get into shape," I'm saying, "Start." Go past "Go." Do anything. Do anything you're willing to do more than once.

If you are like me, you wouldn't go to the gym anyway. Why? "Too much money." "Won't stick with it." "Too embarrassing to work out in public."

Right. I hear all those excuses. They're mine, too. But the bottom line is that you have to start a trend toward fitness. You aren't just burning calories, as good an idea as that is. You are firing up and strengthening your cardiovascular system. You are building and toning muscle, which stimulates metabolism. You are starting a trend toward fitness, and fit bodies resist getting fat.

I hope that on your Fat Days, you'll experiment with walking, jogging, cross-country skiing, biking, swimming, hiking, water aerobics, rowing, jumping rope, spinning, aerobics, and weight training. If you'll work with one or more of these on your Fat Days, you'll find something you'll like, and you'll start to feel stronger.

Outside is always better than inside, but if you have to exercise inside, you have a wonderful list of options. Try the treadmill, an aerobic rider, stair climber, step/ladder climber, an elliptical machine, a cross-country ski machine, a stationary bicycle, a rowing machine, or jump on a minitrampoline. Just do something.

FLUSHING THE CARDIO SYSTEM

However you do it, you need aerobic exercise. I call it a cardiovascular flush. Sometimes when I'm doing one of the exercises I just listed, I like to envision my blood surging through my veins, flushing out the junk that might be accumulating on the walls of my veins and arteries. Flush out your system. Raise your heart rate. Sweat. Pant a little. Breathe. Feel the life. Live.

Remember, you are in the steady process of losing weight and improving your chances of being healthy. And if you do what I recommend, you will become increasingly fit.

Again, mix it up. Play racquetball or squash. Go skiing or snowboarding. Play baseball with family or friends. Need a risk? Try field hockey or ice hockey. Go rock climbing. Play tennis or, if you're like me, act as though you're playing tennis.

Go windsurfing, play volleyball, go dancing, play soccer, ride a horse, go water-skiing, play football, or at least throw a football. Go ice-skating, play a round of golf, shoot some baskets, or play a game of basketball with friends. Go to the gym and learn some gymnastics.

So what if you're a hundred pounds overweight and can't do any of those things? It's fine. Just start. You can do more than you've imagined.

Move. Move until you start feeling young again.

Because the Jerusalem Diet is a trajectory-changing diet, you not only lose weight at a steady and healthy pace, but you also lose your tendency to get fat. Many people can lose weight, but if they still have a tendency to get fat because they haven't increased their overall fitness, then their attempts to control their food intake will become frustrating, and they will most likely end up fat again.

With the Jerusalem Diet, you lose the weight and develop a lifestyle of exercise that will tone and build muscle, which means your metabolism will be working for you, your body will be healthier, and you will have lost your tendency to get fat. You will have improved your odds for health.

Change your trajectory. Become healthy. Do it a little at a time, and you'll see results.

CHAPTER 8

A Day on the Jerusalem Diet

In this chapter I'll give an overview of one day on the Jerusalem Diet.

You'll see how easy it can be to incorporate this diet into your life, even if, like me, you have a very full schedule. This is just a template, so you can adjust it to fit your needs. I've already described a few of my days, but I thought you'd enjoy an easy-to-find reference for a typical day of the Jerusalem Diet lifestyle.

You'll also find some useful information on each of the food groups you can eat during the Jerusalem Diet: fruits, vegetables, nuts, and seeds. These types of foods are loaded with nutrients and do all kinds of good things in our bodies. I'll just briefly outline some of their benefits. There are many other great resources where you can learn more about the nutritional benefits of fruits, vegetables, nuts, and seeds and the incredible, seemingly endless benefits of water. I recommend *Eat, Drink, and Be Healthy* by Walter Willett and *Total Nutrition* from the Mount Sinai School of Medicine. Or you can go online and find an abundance of information and materials.

TIME TO GET UP

When I get up in the morning, I get out of bed and use the bathroom. Then I weigh myself. That's always the first step in this diet.

This is where problems start if you have a cheap scale. With the Jerusalem Diet the only expensive investment you should make up-front is a very good digital scale. Why? Because the report from your scale determines what the rest of your day is going to be like.

Remember, if you are above your target weight for the day, you'll eat fruits, vegetables, nuts, and seeds—and drink water. In addition, you'll exercise one hour. If you're on target or below, eat and exercise as you like.

Because we're seeking only a one-pound difference each week, the idea here is that you shouldn't need the fruits, vegetables, nuts, seeds, and water diet on consecutive days. In total you may have a Fat Day a couple of times a week or maybe as seldom as once a month. It depends on you. The frequency of off-target days will depend on many factors, but don't knock yourself out. One pound a week is all we're after.

I know some think one-pound-a-week weight loss is not much, but think of a pound of butter in your refrigerator. You'll have to use the amount of energy stored in that pound of excess weight during a week. In order to do this, you'll need to exercise and eat according to the plan while drinking plenty of water. As you do, you'll lose the weight just fine.

When your body is burning its own fat instead of food, it's no fun. It feels different, but it has to happen. Because of this, you want the measurement of your weight to be accurate, or you'll get unnecessarily discouraged. Even at one pound a week, it's this first measurement in the morning that counts. This is the one that you respond to. This is your benchmark for the day.

If you have reached and are maintaining your ideal weight, you still want this measurement to be accurate. Why? Because if you can sustain a consistent weight at or a few pounds below your ideal weight, that means you have flexibility. It means you can indulge when your friends indulge. So this first weighing is important.

For women, because of your monthly cycle, you will tend to retain water some days of the month. It's all right. Stay steady. Keep with the system. If the scale says you are having a Fat Day, then eat fruits, vegetables, nuts, and seeds, drink water, and spend an hour exercising. It may even help you to feel better on those difficult days.

MORNING SECRET

I don't know where I read it, but years ago I read about three exercises anyone could do in a hotel room or the bedroom. I thought it sounded good, so I decided to incorporate these into my lifestyle.

When I started the Jerusalem Diet, I was too heavy to do these exercises at all. But as I started to lose weight, I took the advice in this article and tried to do these three simple exercises every morning: sit-ups, squats, and push-ups. Pretty simple. It's a great way to start the day. (Of course, if you're quite out of shape, you should check with a doctor before trying new exercises.)

When I mentioned this earlier in the book, I suggested you start this two-thirds of the way between your first week and your ideal weight and build slowly, one set on day one, two on day two, and so on. Need more exercise tips? Check out the "Move Your Body However You Can" chapter.

BREAKFAST

It's important to eat breakfast to kick-start your body for the day and to give you healthy energy. Whether I am having a Fat Day or not, I tend to eat a light breakfast. If it's not a Fat Day, I eat what I want. If I occasionally want a heavy breakfast, I tend toward the Atkins breakfast of eggs and some kind of meat. If I want to eat light, I usually have cereal, fruit, or yogurt. If I'm having a Fat Day, I'll have a variety of fruits, vegetables, nuts, and seeds and drink water. Sometimes I just eat an apple, an orange, or a banana. Other times

I pull out the juicer or blender and make delicious concoctions of fruit or vegetable juices. That's enough for me.

MIDMORNING MUNCHIES

Typically, there are nuts around the office. We plan it that way; it's part of the food culture we've created. My assistant, Meg, buys cans of mixed nuts and cans of cashews. We mix them in a big bowl in the center of our conference table so people can munch during meetings. We have water, soft drinks, coffee, juices, and cans of Arizona tea for people to drink. As I've mentioned, we also have a bowl of Jelly Bellies.

Contrary to the impression I give, I most often eat the nuts. But on occasion, I'll munch on the Jelly Bellies. Sometimes we will have trail mix—usually seeds, nuts, and M&M's—instead of mixed nuts, and people like that a lot. On regular days, anyone can eat whatever they get when they grab a handful. On Fat Days, the M&M's have to go.

LUNCHTIME

Lunch is when you get fuel for the long afternoon stretch until dinner. If you have a very busy schedule, it's easy to skip lunch, but it's never wise. You'll be crabby or at least weakened as the afternoon wears on.

And if you're really interested in losing weight, lunch is crucial so that you don't indulge later. Skip lunch and you'll be famished later, desperate for energy and willing to ingest the closest thing in reach—a muffin, a candy bar, whatever.

Be wise. Eat lunch. Have a salad with good multigrain bread. Fix a big sandwich with fresh meat and lots of veggies. And drink plenty of water to keep you hydrated through the rest of the day.

LUNCHTIME SECRET

If you are going to plunge into the bowels of debauchery with simple carbs or refined sugar, lunch is the time to do it. Seriously. If you are going to poison yourself, midday poison is the best! You'll pay the least for midday indulgences. Why? Because you are up and going. You will be going for the rest of the afternoon and evening, so you won't pay nearly the price that you would pay if you eat junk in the evening.

If you're going to eat fast food, eat it for lunch.

If you are going to Baskin-Robbins for dessert, do it at lunch.

If you are plunging into despair and can only be satisfied with a visit to Krispy Kreme, do it at lunch.

Timing is everything.

Understand, I'm not recommending these foods. I just know we sometimes desire them, and we need to have systems to handle these desires. Look, I think our bodies were built for survival—we can and do handle an awful lot of junk. It's not best, but we can survive. If we moderate junk and time it well, we will be better off.

I suppose I ought to give a disclaimer here. I've been teaching and practicing the principles of the Jerusalem Diet for years. I've enjoyed it, and so have the thousands of others who have joined me. At least half the pleasure of the Jerusalem Diet is that you can indulge in a Banana Royale from the ice-cream store and brag about how it's part of the Jerusalem Diet weight-loss plan.

My friends tell me we ought to have a series of before and after pictures of people who are on the Jerusalem Diet, with the before and after pictures being identical...except that in the before picture the people are sad, and in the after picture they are smiling! Ha! That's the strength of this diet—it makes you happy. It liberates you to enjoy food and enjoy yourself again.

If you are going to eat food that has no redeeming value, do it at lunch.

Hopefully, you'll move enough in the afternoon and evening that you'll rid yourself of the junk and be able to sleep that night without toxins oozing into every cell of your body.

If, on the other hand, you are having a Fat Day, salads are great lunches. Don't be too rigid here. If some of the ingredients in the salad are not fruits, vegetables, nuts, and seeds, don't worry about it. It won't throw you off too much. Use dressing—don't be legalistic about this. And have meat if you must—salmon or chicken salad is great.

Or say it's a Fat Day, and you end up in a Chinese restaurant. Have the vegetable stir-fry. Use brown rice if you can, but don't sweat it too much. If you are in a normal restaurant, have a couple of side orders of vegetables for lunch. Just about every restaurant has something good to eat that more or less fits the Jerusalem Diet for lunch.

MIDAFTERNOON GRAZING

The principle here is the same as midmorning munchies. Obviously, it's great to have orange segments, apple slices, celery, baby carrots, or anything like that around the office or the house so you can graze on them. Add some nuts, and you will feel more satisfied and full.

THE GRAZE-ALL-DAY SECRET

If you are in a weight-loss mode (whether you're having a Fat Day or not), don't starve yourself. Instead, avoid large portions. Eat a small breakfast, graze midmorning, have a wise and light lunch, graze on carrot sticks and nuts in the afternoon, then have a light dinner and yogurt before you go to bed. You will have eaten six times that day. Also remember to drink plenty of water. Exercise for an hour sometime during the day. It's perfect!

I've had a weight problem since I had children and began living on mostly junk food. I cook for my family, but there are always chips and cookies around the house. In October 2004 I had knee surgery and could no longer walk for exercise. I gained *a lot* of weight in the following months.

In February 2005 I weighed myself, and it was the most I've ever weighed. I became very depressed.

Soon after, I heard your Jerusalem Diet teaching. Since I started incorporating the ideas, I've lost twenty-five pounds. I bought a scale. I never used scales before. I didn't want a reminder of how much weight I had gained or how big I was. The scale was a big step, but it has helped me stay on task. Now I know when I need healthier food and when I can have a treat.

I've begun putting fruits, veggies, and nuts out for my family to munch on instead of chips and cookies. This is an adjustment, but we are getting better.

I have much more weight to lose, but the pounds are coming off. I'm making changes to my eating habits. My mind is no longer on food all the time as it was on other diets. I'm actually beginning to choose healthier food. I believe this will be a lifestyle change. The Jerusalem Diet is easier for me because I'm not always denying myself a candy bar or bowl of ice cream. I thank God for his direction and help. And I'm grateful he used you and your idea to help me.

Thanks very much,

Jan

Later I'll explain how your body will release the energy stored in cells if it thinks you are eating, but if it thinks you might be starving, it will hold on to your fat, thinking it might need this energy in the future. Thus, those who starve, then binge, end up fatter than those who eat several average-sized meals.

DINNER

Sometimes when I'm not having a Fat Day but don't want to have one the next day, I'll weigh myself about this time of day to see how much I can eat during dinner and the evening. Typically, I'll be one to two pounds less in the morning. So I'll weigh myself before dinner, and that will indicate how much wiggle room I have before the next morning.

If I'm having a Fat Day, then my dinner and evening plans are set. If I'm eating out, it's fruits, vegetables, nuts, seeds, and water. If I'm at home, we have this same combination but often have some kind of vegetable dish that we use as an entrée. Some evenings I like eating a couple of apples or oranges. A good salad with nuts and seeds on top is also great for dinner. I try to finish dinner by 7:00 and not eat again unless I have a small snack just before bed. Using the 7:00 p.m. rule, I have time and activity before I go to bed, which is good for me.

BEDTIME

I'll often cheat just before bedtime and eat some yogurt. Most yogurt containers are the perfect size, and the yogurt tastes soooo good. Plus they are great for you. A recent WebMD article suggested that yogurt actually aids in weight loss. The article discussed a study outlined in the *International Journal of Obesity* where two groups of people were put on the same diet, but one group was allowed servings of fat-free yogurt. The yogurt group lost 22 percent more weight, 61 percent more body fat, and 81 percent more belly fat. Isn't that incredible? Researchers are concluding that diets that incorporate calcium and protein from low-fat dairy foods promote weight loss.[1]

If I don't have yogurt, I'll often nibble on a piece of fruit before bed, and I almost always drink a full glass of water to cleanse and hydrate my system while I sleep.

CHAPTER 9

Weigh Yourself Daily

E very day starts the same way. Each morning you can find me in the same place—groggily standing on my bathroom scale, anxiously anticipating the number appearing between my feet.

Lots of diet guides shy away from the advice to weigh yourself daily, because they're afraid people will become obsessive about that little number staring up at them every day. I say: choose your obsessions wisely.

Daily routines are important. Some of the most successful people I know in the world of finance talk about the necessity of checking their financial portfolio every day. People of faith talk about the inspiration they maintain if they read their Bibles and pray first thing in the morning. Early morning routines establish the direction of the day.

None of us would hesitate to brush our teeth, shower, and ensure that our clothes and hair are the way they should be for the day. Since our overall health determines not just how we'll look and feel today but how we'll be able to live for years to come, I think it's well worth taking a couple of seconds to step on a scale and give ourselves direction about our diet and exercise for the day. Weighing yourself in the morning simply gives you a plumb line. If you are close to the edge, hold off. If you have lots of room, enjoy!

If there is a fifty-pound gap between where you are and where you want to be, then avoiding the scale may be good advice. If you're on a diet plan that keeps reminding you that you have dozens more pounds to lose, a daily weigh-in will probably be discouraging.

But on the Jerusalem Diet, you are never more than one or two pounds away from a milestone, one or two pounds away from success. The Jerusalem Diet is for people who can be disciplined for only twenty-four hours at a time. And in order to know how disciplined you need to be on any given day, you need to know your weight in the morning.

So, for this diet, I don't think a daily weigh-in is too oppressive. I want you to be familiar with where you are so you can plan your day accordingly. Remember, if you mess up, just roll with the punches and try again the next day. Having a cheeseburger is not the end of the world.

On the other hand, to work off a pound of fat a week, you have to be intentional. It's one thing to burn the calories derived from a bowl of ice cream you ate a couple of hours ago. It's quite another to work off the fat that your body stored long ago. You have to work off the fat stored deep in your body. That means practicing a day of discipline so that you eat an apple and drink water rather than reach for another bowl of ice cream.

I don't want you to have to do that every day, but I want you to do it when you need to. A daily weigh-in will alert you to where you are in your slow, steady progress toward your ideal weight.

YOU ARE WHAT YOU WEIGH

Remember, weight is a great indicator of overall health. Dr. Walter Willett says, "Next to whether you smoke, the number that stares up at you from the bathroom scale is the most important measure of your future health. Keeping that number in the healthy range is more important for long-term health than the types and amounts of antioxidants in your food or the exact ratio of fats to carbohydrates."[1] I love his take on this, because it puts in context all the cultural dieting hysteria over carbs, low-fat meals, and antioxidants. Willett is saying, "Sure, sure, that's all great. But what do you weigh?"

Furthermore, Willett explains that one way to guess your current level of fitness is to consider how much your waist has grown since your early twenties. What size pants were you wearing in college or in that first professional job? How many notches have you gained on your belt since then?

If this line of thinking discourages you, keep your chin up. It should be clear by now that my goal for this diet is total well-being. Even if you have a long way to go to achieve your ideal weight, your weekly target weight should never be too far out of reach. If you're at your target weight on any given week in the Jerusalem Diet, then by all means, the number staring up at you from the scale is no big deal, even if it is a big number. Just let it drop one pound at a time, at a pace you can live with. Change your life slowly.

But as you're changing your life, be familiar with what needs to change. Weigh yourself daily—just as a plumb line. Don't get upset if, rather than lose weight, you gain a pound or a few or have a long plateau. I just want you to have an idea of where you are so you can plan your days accordingly.

How to Weigh Yourself

The daily weigh-in is something you need to be consistent about. Do it at the same time every day with a similar amount of clothes (or no clothes) on. Don't do it while dripping wet or even if just your hair is wet—that'll increase the number for sure. Do it after going to the rest room and before eating. For me, the easiest time is first thing in the morning. Some people say you don't get an accurate weight in the morning, because your weight adjusts as the day goes on. That's true, which is why you need to weigh at the same time each day.

Pay attention to this idea. If you are random with this, the Jerusalem Diet will be hit and miss, and you'll be disappointed.

Don't forget, we want to achieve our ideal weight and stay there. Your target weight is the daily goal you use while losing weight, declining by one pound a week. Your ideal weight is the weight at which you will be most comfortable—the weight you want to achieve and maintain.

By the way, if you are one of those needing to gain weight, reverse the process. When you are below weight, you should do exercises that build muscle, and you should drink and eat the types of food that will help you gain weight. There are many resources available to help you. I suggest you visit a GNC dealer or check with a Shaklee or Quixtar dealer to get the guidance you need for weight gain.

Getting a Handle on Those Handles

One of the most surprising things about weighing yourself every day is that your weight probably fluctuates more than you think. You may not know how inconsistent your eating patterns are and how much they are affecting your weight. You also may not know how much water retention and gastrointestinal content can affect what you see on the scale. Getting into the habit of seeing that number every day, at about the same time every day, will make you more familiar with what's going on in your body. In time you'll eat with full knowledge of how it will affect the next day's weigh-in.

If I'm teetering just under my target weight, I know that the decisions I make in the middle of the afternoon may affect what I see on the scale the next morning. As I've said, sometimes the thought of a huge waffle cone of rocky road ice cream is just too delicious, so I enjoy it even though I know it means that tomorrow I may have only fruits, vegetables, nuts, and seeds with water and exercise.

I like this familiarity with my weight. I like knowing the consequences of what I eat, rather than letting it remain a mystery. I find it much more enjoyable and helpful to work with full knowledge than to have no clue what's happening inside me.

More than anything else, the daily weigh-in has helped me have confidence. Being consistent about weighing myself has made me more flexible in my eating habits. I know when I can eat whatever I want, and I know that even when I can't, it won't take me long to get back on target. Sometimes on your fruits, vegetables, nuts, seeds, and water days, you might sneak a piece of cheesecake. You are forgiven. Because the next day you'll weigh yourself, and you'll find out the consequences. Maybe you'll get away with something. Or maybe you'll learn how little you can get away with. Either way, you're better off knowing than not knowing.

HOW TO BE OKAY WHEN YOU CAN'T WEIGH

Right now I am traveling, and I don't have a scale with me. I've learned that there are three choices while traveling:

1. Get fat.
2. Try to discipline what you eat in general so you don't gain too much weight.
3. Curb your appetite and get even a little exercise.

I've done all of these things. My favorite is number 3. Here is how I do it.

As you know, on the Jerusalem Diet, there are no required supplements, though if you want to use supplements, there are natural/herbal products available at health-food stores that can be helpful. When I'm traveling, since I can't weigh myself every morning, I take nutritional supplements and drink a lot of water to help curb my appetite. That way, when I get home, I'm usually at or near my target weight. I know from experience how discouraging it can be to come home several pounds overweight. It feels great to get home from a trip and be right on or even below target.

While we're on the subject of traveling, let me encourage you to exercise a little more while traveling. I always pack exercise clothes and find that it's wonderful to take a walk, go for a jog, or go swimming. You don't have to press hard; just enjoy using your muscles to tone them a little. If, however, you like to lift weights, you might have more free time than at home, so press hard and let the travel time be a time to exercise, eat right, drink plenty of water, and rest.

Bottom line for this chapter: Weigh yourself daily. It will provide the plumb line to keep you on track.

CHAPTER 10

Eat Fat-Day Foods

B y now you know, if you weigh yourself and find that you're a pound or more overweight, don't throw the scale out the window. Don't go on a two-week fast or try some gimmicky diet that only lets you eat alfalfa sprouts.

Instead, just have a Fat Day.

Remember, on the Jerusalem Diet, a Fat Day isn't a day where you are actually fat. It's just a day where you are over your target weight for the day. It's a day when you probably feel a little heavier because you enjoyed a greasy pork sandwich and chocolate-chip sundae the day before. But it's no big deal. It's just a Fat Day, and after eating fruits, vegetables, nuts, and seeds, drinking water, and doing an hour of exercise, you'll be back on target tomorrow.

Fat Days are not bad days. But in case you need extra convincing to get you through them, I wanted to include a chapter that would give you some specifics about all the great stuff you're doing to your body on Fat Days. (Don't you love it—on the Jerusalem Diet, Fat Days are the most nutritional days of all!)

BE FRUIT FULL!

Hardly anyone needs convincing to eat fruit, of course, but how adventurous are you in your fruit selection? Have you realized how many different, delicious ways there are to make your diet more fruit full? The produce section in your supermarket has undergone a revolution in recent years. Fruits that were once considered exotic can now be found in any grocery store. When I was an adolescent, the average market contained around 65 different fresh produce items. By the early eighties, that number had nearly tripled to 173 items. Some larger stores may have as many as 250 items.[1] Today, whether I walk into a store emphasizing organic foods or a regular grocery, I can find a wide range of both organic and conventionally grown fruits, all of which are nutritious and delicious. We're living in Eden again!

As a result of a busy schedule, maybe you take a vitamin C and let that suffice for your fruit quotient each day. This is better than nothing, but it doesn't replace the real thing. Many companies offer supplements in pill form that are the best that fruit has to offer, but those supplements still aren't actual fruit. For example, setting aside the fact that citrus fruit does a lot more for the body than provide a dose of vitamin C, those tablets can't replace fruit as a source of the vitamin. Why? Because citrus fruit contains two forms of vitamin C—ascorbic acid and dehydroascorbic acid—and both are necessary to get C's full power potential. Don't take my word for it; the Mount Sinai School of Medicine's nutrition guide, *Total Nutrition,* reports this. Eating fruit is the only way to get a balanced supply of an essential vitamin like C.

The U.S. Department of Health and Human Services recommends you eat five servings of fruit a day, making sure that you eat a wide range so you can get all the benefits in fruit, from vitamins A and C to fiber and beta carotene. Other groups and programs recommend as many as nine servings of fruits and vegetables. Bottom line: you won't overeat on fruits and vegetables.

I think research is going to increasingly demonstrate unexpected benefits of eating real (as opposed to processed or pill-form) food like fruit. For example, not long ago *Family Practice News* reported that increased fruit in the diet of African Americans decreased hypertension. Here's a summary of this research:

Aware of clinical studies showing the benefits of the Dietary Approaches to Stop Hypertension (DASH), Kristie J. Lancaster, Ph.D., set out to assess dietary patterns and blood pressure levels among African Americans in a free-living community.

She and her associates evaluated a sample of 4,732 African Americans aged 25 years and older who provided 24-hour dietary recall information as part of the National Health and Nutrition Examination Survey III.

After adjustment for age and body mass index, higher fruit intake was associated with lower systolic blood pressures in both men and women. More fruit servings also were associated with lower diastolic blood pressures in women.[2]

This is just one example of tons of research that is telling us the same thing: eat fruit. Don't try to get by with only using supplements or drinking juices. You were made to munch. Eat the real stuff.

Just keep fruit around the house and office, and make your selection as colorful as possible. As a rule of thumb, the more colors of fruit you eat, the more nutritional benefit you get. Fruits contain varieties of phytochemicals that have different antioxidants and nutrients, which perform different healthy functions in our bodies. Blueberries, in particular, have an abundance of antioxidants. (I've heard rumors that blueberries affect some men like Viagra! That might be an unwarranted rumor. But why not try it? Women, get your husbands to eat more blueberries!) Oranges and apricots have loads of vitamin A. Apples, strawberries, mangoes, grapefruit, passionfruit, bananas—the colorful spectrum of these fruits represents a whole range of benefits they offer. Keep your fruit selection colorful and plentiful.

Let fruit be part of the food culture of your home. In the summertime we like to imitate the tropics—bunches of bananas, stacks of pineapple slices, papayas, mangoes, and oranges. Add to this, berries, cherries, grapes, peaches, and plums. I like grapefruit in the morning, preferably in juice form.

Fruits are also a great substitute for desserts, and you can even be a little decadent with them. Check out this good news from *Total Nutrition* about using fruits as desserts:

> Fruits are often suggested as a low-fat dessert, but their possibilities in this department go beyond the raw fruit eaten out of hand. Fruits such as pears and plums can be poached in a very light syrup; berries and other juicy fruits can be whipped with yogurt or pectin into frappés— or spreads, or used to flavor water ices and low-fat sherbets; fruit juices can be frozen into Popsicles or cubes, or mixed with gelatin, to provide a treat for children. While many such preparations may have significant amounts of natural or added sugar, their big advantage over commercial baked goods and other desserts is their lack of saturated fat.[3]

I love this, because it introduces another variable into our eating habits. There are so many ways to prepare and enjoy fruit, and if, like me, you have a sweet tooth (or a whole set of sweet teeth), you can find ways to satisfy that craving while getting all the nutritious benefits of fruit. People will tell you, "If you don't eat fruit totally raw, you aren't doing yourself any good." Don't listen to them. Find as many ways as you like to prepare and eat fruits.

What about shopping for fruits? Well, if you're following the color principle, just load your basket with as much color as possible. Fruits are always best and most affordable when they're in season, and there's nothing wrong with letting the time of year determine your fruit-eating habits— berries in late spring and summer, apples in the fall. Pile fruit on your counter or table until it ripens, then let it keep in the refrigerator. But once it's chilling in the fridge, don't let fruit overstay its welcome. During a long stay in the crisper, fruit will eventually lose taste and nutrient levels.[4]

Fresh fruit is always best, but don't shy away from frozen versions, because there is little difference in terms of nutrient levels. The *Total Nutrition* guide notes, "Freezing is actually one of the least destructive methods of food preservation available."[5] Likewise, dried fruit has about the same amount of vitamins and nutrients, but it can increase your calorie intake—since there's no water, you have to eat more to feel full.

The main thing is to keep fruit around—and, again, keep it colorful.

EAT A GARDEN!

People split hairs over the differences between fruits and vegetables, and nuts and seeds. Technically, "vegetables" such as tomatoes are actually fruits, and some nuts and seeds fit into the fruit category. A fruit is the ripened, seed-bearing ovary of a plant or tree, and a vegetable is the root or leafy, tuber, or stalk part of a plant. But for clarity's sake, let's call vegetables those things in the produce section of your grocery store that you know aren't fruits. For you and me, it's best to stick with those grocery-store groupings and let tomatoes, cucumbers, eggplants, avocados, corn, and other fruits be what they've always been to us: good vegetables.

Like fruits, vegetables improve energy, protect eyesight, stimulate digestive health, and provide defense against diseases such as cancer. They are a primary source of many vitamins, minerals, and antioxidants, and they are low in fat and cholesterol. As with fruits, the U.S. government recommends that Americans consume at least five servings of vegetables each day.

Vegetables are like preventive medicine: they can reduce your chances of a heart attack and stroke, lower your blood pressure, and, again, protect against cancer. Vegetables fight cataracts and macular degeneration, two common eye diseases. And as with fruits, you can't get away with eating the same kinds of vegetables all the time. Here again, color is key: the more varied the palette of your vegetable intake, the better the health benefit to your body.

Why is this the case? Why can't you just eat a small variety of vegetables or, better yet, get your nutrients in pill form? Call it the great unknown factor. We know a lot about what vegetables do in our bodies, but there is much not yet known. Plants are responsible for many good things that happen in the human body, because of the phytochemicals they contain. In *Eat, Drink, and Be Healthy,* Dr. Walter Willett reminds us that many—probably most—of these phytochemicals have not yet been discovered. In the near future we may learn that the cancer-fighting, nutrient-providing work vegetables do results from specific qualities we currently haven't identified or from a commingling of qualities.[6] In short, while we know vegetables do an incredible amount of good in our bodies, we don't yet know all the specifics. We can't isolate which vegetable or exactly which aspect of each vegetable has the benefit, so we're better off eating as many kinds as we can as often as we can.

Another reason for variety: we know that vegetables fight cancer, but we also know that it takes different vegetables to fight different kinds of cancers. Broccoli works against bladder cancer, carrots probably work against breast cancer, raw and green vegetables against colon cancer, leafy vegetables against lung cancer, tomatoes against prostate cancer, and so on.[7] Also, the Mount Sinai School of Medicine guide notes that vegetarians have lower blood-pressure levels because of all the great stuff they get from their foods: potassium, magnesium, polyunsaturated fats, vegetable protein, and fiber. People with high vegetable diets have a lower risk of osteoporosis, kidney stones, gallstones, and adult-onset diabetes.

One reason Fat Days are so superb is that as we focus on eating vegetables, we provide our bodies with essential dietary fiber. This is no small thing. Fiber is the part of fruits, vegetables, nuts, and seeds that we can't digest; it aids in keeping our systems regular and our blood cholesterol manageable. Having enough dietary fiber might just save your life—it aids in protecting the heart against coronary heart diseases such as stroke and heart attack.

Eat your vegetables. Don't just drink them or take them in pill form. You need to eat them and receive all the life-giving benefits they offer. However, pills are better than nothing, and the real thing is better than pills.

Like fruits, vegetables are best fresh and in season. They keep most of their nutrients even in the freezing process, so don't shy away from the packaged varieties. If they are fresh, they should be washed under running water rather than soaked; very dirty vegetables can be scrubbed or cleaned with water.

For vegetables with skin (which is to say, those vegetables that are really fruits, such as cucumbers and tomatoes), most of the nutrients are in the skin. A tomato skin contains three times more vitamin C than the flesh.[8] Try cooking with the peel still on the vegetable, even if you want to remove it before serving. Same goes for leaves—the leafy ends of lettuce, cabbage, kale, collard greens, and turnip greens are the most nutritious, just as broccoli's best stuff is on the leaf rather than in the stalks or florets. Cook it all to make sure you're getting the full benefit. And eat your parsley—it's not just a garnish but a nutrient-rich vegetable.

In general, the more you cook a vegetable, the less good you're getting from it. Stir-fry or steaming is best; boiling and stewing is worst. But eat 'em any way you will.

GO NUTS!

Nuts are, by truest definition, seeds. They are little balls of plant DNA, the building blocks for trees and shrubs and many other types of plant. What differentiates nuts from other seeds is the hard shell in which the kernel rests.

Nuts are a great part of a daily diet, and as a healthy protein package, they are definitely a great replacement for meat during your twenty-four-hour adjustment. Does that mean you should fire up the grill and throw on a pound of cashews? No. But used sensibly, nuts can provide you with tons of nutritional benefits and help you lose weight if you need to.

About a decade ago, nuts were written off by many dietitians because of their high fat content and high calories. However, certain fats, many of which are contained in nuts, have recently been put back on the good-for-you list. The body needs essential ("essential" means you need to ingest it; your body will not produce it) fats, including omega-3 and omega-6 fatty acids. Likewise, most of us require a minimal amount of cholesterol; our hormones, skin, and the membranes of our cells use cholesterol as a building block in their basic structure and production.

In other words, nuts are smart. They have a high fat content, but their fat is mostly unsaturated. They reduce LDL cholesterol (the bad kind) and maintain HDL cholesterol (the good kind). There is a negligible difference in the fat content between nuts roasted in oil and dry-roasted nuts, so eat whichever you like.[9] If you need some historical reason to eat what you eat, nuts are right up your alley. The Romans considered nuts the food of the gods. The Incas made pottery to resemble the highly prized peanut. According to a manuscript from 2838 BC found in China, the hazelnut took its place among the five sacred nourishments bestowed on human beings. Walnuts were prescribed for head ailments during the Renaissance.

Nuts are known to help fight cancer and reduce the risk of heart disease. They are a good source of protein, fiber, minerals, vitamins B and E, and several good dietary fats. Most are sold as sources of B vitamins and iron.[10] People who include nuts as a regular part of their diet are 25–39 percent less likely to contract coronary artery disease.[11]

Nuts are a great snack, and peanuts in quantity are still better than candy. Several clinical studies also support the heart-healthy benefits of nuts. In 1993 a paper published in the *New England Journal of Medicine* demonstrated that substituting a percentage of walnuts for other fatty foods in the diet reduced serum cholesterol by more than 10 percent in the men who participated in the study. Again, lowering cholesterol means improving overall heart health and reducing the risk of heart disease. The researchers agree that more work needs to be done, but they believe prudent nut consumption is beneficial.[12]

As Steven Pratt emphasizes in *SuperFoods Rx,* "All nuts and seeds are significant contributors to your good health. It makes sense that nuts and seeds are rich sources of a wide variety of nutrients. They are, after all, nature's nurseries. A nut or seed is basically a storage device that contains all the highly concentrated proteins, calories, and nutrients that a plant embryo will require to flourish."[13]

Of the four food types you must eat while you are enjoying your twenty-four-hour Jerusalem Diet, nuts should be used most sparingly. Because they are high in fat, the recommended dose per day is 1.5 ounces—that's about a handful. Don't eat so many nuts that you obliterate their benefits. But a handful of nuts is a fantastic and healthy way to cut hunger, and nuts can be a great part of main dishes, such as pad Thai and some Asian and Mediterranean cuisine. And even a few nuts are filling, which is why I use them to replace meat on my Fat Days. Remember, walnuts are on the superfood list, so I buy walnuts in bulk to munch on. But you should eat whatever tastes good and work toward healthier choices from there.

Not Just for Sowing

Seeds are no longer just for road trips, baseball games, and making luscious gardens. I love to add seeds to my salad at lunch. They are a great stir-fry addition for the evening meal, and lots of recipes use seeds to add flavor and crunchiness as well as substantial health benefits.

Medical research continues to uncover the power-packed nature of this small food group. According to the Food and Drug Administration, any food with 20 percent or more of the daily value for a nutrient is considered an "excellent" source of that nutrient. Therefore, sunflower, sesame, pumpkin, and many other seeds are "excellent" sources for a handful of nutrients such as protein, vitamin E, copper, and zinc.

Your body stores many things, but protein isn't one of them. You have to put it in. Protein's main task is to supply the body with amino acids, which are the foundation of building, maintaining, and repairing body tissue and protecting bones, muscles, cartilage, skin, and blood. Seeds are a protein-heavy food. Just a handful of sunflower seeds provides the body with more than six grams of protein, or nearly one-fifth of the daily requirement. There is some fat with that protein, but nearly 90 percent of the fat in sunflower seeds is good, unsaturated fat.

Sunflower seeds are also the best-known whole food source of vitamin E. One ounce provides the body with more than 75 percent of the daily requirement. Risks such as heart disease and prostate cancer are lowered with a healthy preventative dose of vitamin E. This is because vitamin E aids in ridding the body of harmful molecules called free radicals, which can lead to certain cancers and diseases like atherosclerosis.

Some seeds carry 25–75 percent of the daily requirements of copper. Sesame seeds have the highest concentration of copper, which helps the body carry oxygen to red blood cells. Copper also helps produce energy within the cells. Just like vitamin E, copper helps to protect the body from the damage caused by free radicals. It also helps to protect against heart disease and strokes and is good for both the immune and skeletal systems.

Of the seed family, pumpkin seeds contain the highest concentration of zinc, at 25 percent of the daily requirement from a one-ounce serving. Zinc is essential for maintaining strength in the immune system. Research has shown that diets complete with the full daily requirement of zinc help keep the prostate healthy. In addition to zinc, dried pumpkin seeds are packed with magnesium, manganese, and phosphorus.

Seeds contain many other nutrients as well, including folate, iron, and fiber. Folate, another B vitamin, plays an essential role in cell reproduction and may help prevent heart disease. Iron plays a crucial role in carrying oxygen from your lungs to your cells. An iron deficiency typically leads to fatigue and infection. Fiber, which helps lower cholesterol, manages blood glucose and helps prevent constipation.

Treat seeds as you would nuts—keep them around in bowls for snacking and add them to other meals. I often buy a package of seeds and eat them as I drive or as I wait in airports. On your Fat Days, you'll find that they are a great way to curb your appetite and keep you going throughout the day.

I want to thank you for the Jerusalem Diet! I went to the health and fitness meeting you had, and it felt so good. I bought a juicer and a good scale, and I love them both very much. When I started the diet, I weighed 258.6 pounds. This morning I was at 243…and my target for today is just 247.6!

I had given up on losing any weight. I tried all the programs, just as you said your mom did, and none of them worked. I would only be able to keep up for a couple of weeks. I lost the same fifteen pounds over and over again! I still struggle with emotional eating from time to time, but that is getting better each week.

My whole approach to eating has changed. I have taken what I learned from all the other programs and added it to this one. I'm eating the correct portions (most of the time) and eating more healthy food. The binging has all but stopped! This has been such a great experience for me, and I finally have the hope that I will be fit and healthy so I can live a full life!

Thanks again,

Debbie

THE DIETER'S FRIEND

It's too bad that water is sometimes associated with being overweight; often you'll hear women talk about wanting to lose their "water weight." Of course, in certain times they do have water pounds to shed, but drinking less water isn't the answer. Your body needs plenty of fluid for you to be fit. And of all the fluids available today—from lattes to fruit drinks to (yes) Mountain Dew—water is far and away the best.

You see, water makes your body work. Like putting oil in your engine and gas in your tank, water is the lubricant that keeps your parts running smoothly and efficiently.

Think about your metabolism. Your body metabolizes fat for energy. All the talk about efficient or inefficient, active or slow metabolism is really about how well a body breaks down fat into usable energy. Water is an important key to your body's metabolizing functions—your body needs fluid to help break down fat.

I know drinking lots of water can make you feel full or bloated and therefore trick you into thinking it's not good for weight loss. But even if it makes you feel full, your body needs water. And that full feeling has an additional benefit: it's a cure for the munchies. If you find yourself craving a sugary muffin for a midafternoon snack, gulp down a bottle of water instead. It's a calorie-free way to curb your appetite.

Of course, water isn't technically a weight-loss tool; it just does tons of good things for our bodies. It regulates body temperature, removes toxins and wastes, and lubricates our joints. It carries nutrients and oxygen to our cells. Water is easy for the body to absorb and easy for the body to flush.

How much water should you drink? Drink a glass with meals, and drink some between meals. You've probably heard that we all need eight glasses a day, which is a standard many people use, though some argue for less. Milk, juice, and other drinks and foods contain water too, so if you're trying for a certain number of glasses, they don't all have to be actual water. But water is the best option.

One way to gauge your water intake is to pay attention to the color of your urine. Remember, pee pale. If your urine is dark yellow or smelly, you probably are dehydrated and need to drink more water. If it is totally clear, you can hold off. But keep the water coming in, and your body will keep your system running smoothly.

Fruits. Vegetables. Nuts. Seeds. Water. These are your Fat Day foods and beverage. Enjoy!

CHAPTER 11

Move Your Body However You Can

I feel great today! Yesterday I went jogging in Vail, Colorado, and it was beautiful. I was on a trail that runs alongside a picturesque mountain stream rushing with fresh snowmelt. It was gorgeous.

Remember, I'm forty-nine years old without any genetic advantages. According to the odds, I should be arthritic, overweight, and diabetic. Instead, I'm healthy, able to run and breathe deeply, and I love life.

Yesterday was Saturday, and since we were enjoying a minibreak in the mountains, I woke up slowly. While still lying in bed, my wife read aloud four chapters from Ephesians, one of my favorite books of the Bible. When I got up, I did my push-ups, sit-ups, and squats. Then I rested while reading the paper, and next I went for a run. When I got back, I ate some fruit over cottage cheese while catching up on phone calls and e-mails. I wrote for a while. Then I had a massage. We ate salmon for dinner, watched a movie together, read for an hour, and went to bed.

While I was getting my massage, I discussed health with the massage therapist. In response to one of his comments, I told him about the oldest man I'd ever met. He is a pastor in Lagos, Nigeria, and is 114 years old. When he was a boy, he lied about his age in order to fight in World War I. He had outlived four wives, had hundreds of grandchildren, and was one of the most happy, spunky, lucid, and exciting men I'd ever met. He had strong opinions about the current geopolitical situation and was a supporter of American involvement in policing the world. He was feisty. When I met with him, he was getting ready to speak to sixty thousand people! He was incredible.

Of course I wanted to know to what he attributed his health and longevity. I started by asking him if he liked Coke. He laughed and said that he did, in fact. Then I asked how he explained his long life and bright mind.

He said that he read or had others read to him every day and that he discussed new ideas with people every day. Every day he exercised, and now that he was 114, that meant stretching. And he said he had a vibrant, Bible-based relationship with God.

I told him that I know lots of people who did all those things, but they were not like him. Then he told me what he really thought.

"I think more people die every day from eating too much rather than from eating too little," he said. "I eat two meals a day and munch a little in between. That's it."

Understand, this man is from Lagos, which means that his meals have been more natural than ours would likely be, and his "munching" probably hasn't been on processed sugary snacks but on more nutritious snacks. (Hmmmm. Just like the Jerusalem Diet recommends.)

As you can tell from how I spent yesterday, I want to model the life of that pastor. I want to live to be 114 too.

Okay, I know some of you are thinking that you can't live the way I've described. Massages? Running by mountain streams?

My response is, why not? Start adjusting your weight and your activity level, strengthen your spiritual life, read good books that will inform your thinking and discussions with others, and your life will prosper. There's no reason your life cannot improve.

SURROUNDED BY MOTIVATION

Working where I do, I find it pretty easy to be motivated to exercise. There are a bunch of young men and women walking around New Life Church who look as if they are competing for the title of Perfect Human Specimen. Our internship program for high-school graduates, Twenty-four Seven, is led by Christopher Beard, a man whose mission in life is to get young people in shape—spiritually, emotionally, intellectually, and, yes, physically. Christopher makes these poor eighteen- to twenty-two-year-olds get up with the sun every morning and run, bike, and swim their way to health. It's great for teaching discipline and the importance of working through pain and discomfort.

And because most of them end up looking like Olympic athletes, it's also great for motivating me to work out whether I feel like it or not. On days when I'm feeling fat and lazy, one of these kids will walk by, flash me a toothy smile, and say, "Good morning, Pastor Ted!" and all I can think is, *Oh, I hate this! Man, I need to workout!* No matter what else is going on that day, I'll clear some time in my schedule to get my pathetic body on the treadmill, on a bike, or in the pool, or at least do some push-ups. Then I feel better.

As I noted earlier, last summer I ran quite a bit with a twenty-one-year-old friend named Daniel. I always insisted that he let me set the pace, but running with such a young guy pushed me. It seemed Daniel could go forever, smiling the whole time. I felt as if I were a (very slow) greyhound and Daniel was the mechanical rabbit. It was wonderful motivation to get into shape.

Our church's college pastor, Aaron Stern, took me on a run recently that I'm sure added years to my life (or maybe took them off). He encouraged me to do better, not by what he was saying, but simply by running with me.

Two summers ago I asked Christopher to take me to the gym with him and train me the way he would one of his student interns. He declined to do that, saying that he loved me too much. But he did offer to work with me a couple of hours a day. Normally, I don't have that kind of time, but it happened that I'd decided not to travel for about twelve weeks and had three mornings a week to meet Christopher at 24-Hour Fitness. He had me in the best shape I've ever been in. I didn't keep it, but it was incredible. And you know what? It didn't hurt. It was fun. And I'm confident that my body is better off because of that time I spent with Christopher.

More than likely you are not between eighteen and twenty-two years old, and you may not have the advantage of being constantly motivated by Perfect Human Specimens. But look around and notice people. Don't judge them, but do observe them. You'll notice some who are excessive in taking care of themselves. Avoid that. You'll notice others who are healthy and toned. That's where you want to be. You'll notice others who are on the way to obesity. They should motivate you to switch directions. You'll notice some who are simply overweight. Let the overweight ones motivate you as much as those who are in great shape.

How I Move However I Can

I challenge you to seize every opportunity to move your body.

- Park at the outer edge of the parking lot and walk.
- Use the stairs instead of taking the elevator.
- Get in the pool and move in the water.
- Ski and snowboard in the winter.
- Ride your bike.
- Walk with your spouse or a friend in the mornings or evenings.

Any movement is better than just sitting. With that in mind, let me say two things about exercise: (1) No health plan is complete without regular exercise, and (2) you don't have to be an athlete to improve your health.

Whatever else you do for your health, you need to incorporate some

My husband and I have tried many different dieting methods without success. I work forty-plus hours a week, and my husband works twelve-hour days three to four days a week. With our energy levels so low and the fact that we are "not as young as we used to be" (sixty-one and fifty-three), diets that require special cooking and calculating just didn't work. It seemed so hopeless.

In January a doctor suggested I have gastric bypass surgery. That scared me so much.… My husband needed to lose a hundred pounds too.

The Jerusalem Diet has given us hope. We are learning to eat the right kinds of food. We have more energy and are on our way to our weight-loss goals. We increase our exercise every day, and when we aren't getting the results we need, we do more. I ride my exercise bike in the morning before I get ready for work. I have worked up to two miles in eight minutes. I don't have time for much more, but I hope to do better than that.

Weighing every day has been the biggest help. Even though I tend to fluctuate a couple of pounds from day to day, the diet has given me motivation to be diligent. We still go out to eat with friends and family on Sundays and enjoy old favorites, such as steak and baked potatoes, but we watch how much we have.

Our desires have actually been changing. We are more likely to eat the best of what is offered and stay away from fattening foods. We feel free, free, free! We laugh about how good vegetables are and how we'd rather have them than cake or pie. But the bottom line is that we feel free to eat what is available and what we have time to fix. It's a matter of choices. For the first time we feel we can make this a lifelong change.

Pauline and Jim

exercise for your heart and your overall well-being. Nutrition is important, but you have to exercise too. You were not created to be immobile. Your body is a brilliant creation, and it will take care of itself if you stretch it out and work it out. If you don't, you'll suffer. Your cardiovascular system needs stimulation on a regular basis to keep your heart healthy. If you exercise, you'll feel better, be happier, and probably live longer. You'll also lose weight much, much faster than you will without exercising (in part because your metabolism will burn more calories to support increasing muscle mass), so if that's a primary goal for you, exercise is all the more essential.

But what if you're a fat slob? Sorry, but let's face facts. If you don't know a gym sock from a jelly doughnut, getting started is the hardest part. What if you haven't been too far off the sofa for the last decade? What if the most exercise you ever get is reaching for the remote? How do you go from slob to slim?

My answer is the title of this chapter: *move your body however you can.* If the thought of putting on gym shorts and running three miles terrifies you, don't do it. Just begin wherever you are. If you are so immobile that all you can do is bounce in the pool for an hour, do it. Whatever you can do, do it.

Walk down the block. Slightly crouch down and stand up over and over. Lift your arms over your head. Do something. Do something that you won't mind doing again tomorrow and the next day and the day after that. *The best exercise is whatever you will actually do.*

You can buy a set of DVDs by a supermodel; you can buy expensive exercise equipment; you can buy protein supplements and anything else you think will help you get on the fast track to health. Whatever will motivate you helps, but you have to move. Start doing exercise that you don't mind doing. You don't have to run a marathon. You don't even have to walk a mile. Just start by doing whatever you can, however you can.

If you've not exercised in a long time, you will be surprised at the rapid gains that can be made, especially in the first few days and weeks. Your muscles will thank you by being sore, which is a sign that you've created little tears that are healing and making your muscles more fit. Your head will be clearer. You'll be in a better mood. You'll be nicer to your spouse, your kids, and others around you. You'll be a better person.

Health experts say that if you can raise your heart rate for twenty minutes or so per day, you're doing pretty well. On the Jerusalem Diet, you don't have to exercise every day, though of course it's best if you do exercise regularly. But to stick to the diet, all you have to do is one hour of exercise on Fat Days.

It's fine to divide your hour if you like. Walk for twenty minutes. Get into the pool and move for thirty minutes, then walk for another ten minutes. Split up your hour if you need to. Exercising for a solid hour would be best, but for some people that's a target to work toward. If all you can do is a few minutes, then try to do a few minutes a few times a day until you reach an hour. You can split it up any way you want to. The point is that you just need to expend some energy.

You are alive. You are not dead. Your life has value and purpose that can only be fulfilled if you take care of yourself. Today, start moving.

CHAPTER 12

Women and the Jerusalem Diet

by Gayle Haggard

I once heard someone say (who could it have been?) that the absolute best exercise, the one that will benefit you the most, is simply the one you'll do. It doesn't matter if a particular exercise program or machine guarantees that it will take inches off in four weeks. If it is not an exercise that fits into your lifestyle—one that you're comfortable with or that you enjoy doing—you probably won't do it. The guarantee is worthless to you.

The same is true with finding a diet. There is a multitude of diets that promise to help you lose weight or make you healthier, and many of them really do have benefits and work for those who do them. But the best diet is simply the one you'll do.

As I've matured (a nice way of saying it), I've tried many of the popular diets to ward off the results of decreased activity. The keyword here is *tried*. My commitment to them has been only temporary—either because they were difficult to maintain with my lifestyle or because I simply grew weary of them.

I can testify that they all worked for a season, but I never wanted to stick with any of them for life. However, with each diet I've grown a little more educated as to what I like and what I don't like, what I'll do and what I won't do. Thus each of these diets has made a contribution to the diet I can live with—the one I'll do.

Ted has asked me to share a few tips that have helped me along my diet journey. The following is my "body philosophy"—the perspective that helps me live in peace and joy within my body.

ACCEPT YOUR BODY

Probably the most beneficial thing I've learned is to accept my body and be grateful for it. If each of us will take a moment to think about what is good and right about our bodies, we'll find a lot to be grateful for. Can you see your feet, walk, move your arms, smile? Isn't that great?

I think the most beautiful women are those who accept their bodies, are comfortable in their own skin, and make the most of who they are today. When we are able to do this, we won't be so self-focused and can turn our attention and energies outward toward others. We can be loving, kind, and considerate, which are the truest beauty traits.

On the other hand, women who are consumed with how they look—every pound, wrinkle, or flaw—work too hard at perfection and unknowingly become increasingly uninteresting and ugly in the eyes of others.

So the first step is to accept your body and begin to see it as your tool to serve and care for others. Make the most of it, care for it, make it healthy and strong, adorn it beautifully and respectably, and you'll be a long way toward achieving the kind of admiration in the eyes of others—particularly your loved ones—that you desire. And you can be happy in the process!

I think simplicity is the most notable quality of the Jerusalem Diet. It's easy. It doesn't make our lives and the lives of those around us miserable. We can take care of ourselves and enjoy the process, which frees us to be happy and contribute to the happiness of others. Contrast this with being bound up day after day, thinking about ourselves, our weight, every calorie, every failure—making others our enemies when they just want us to relax and have fun. What a miserable way to spend our lives.

BE GENTLE TO YOUR BODY

Once we can accept our bodies and be grateful for what is right about them, we can begin to really care for them. This leads to my second tip: be gentle to your body.

This means to work with your body, not against it. Find out what foods and eating patterns work best for your body, what exercises you can do and enjoy doing, how to balance rest with work, and how much sleep you really need. I call this "peace to your body," and I believe it is the best form of preventive medicine.

Current beauty standards would have us abuse our bodies by starving them, exercising them to the point of pain or severe discomfort, or using artificial and extreme supplementation to shed pounds, gain muscle, or lose body fat. They also encourage invasive measures to obtain a sleek figure. Be careful—there can be harmful side effects and results.

I understand that there are times when severe circumstances call for severe measures. But we cannot live our lives going from one severe measure to another. This requires too much self-focus, and it is a miserable way to live. Instead, why not be gentle to your body and work with it in the way it was designed to work best?

Remember the old adages "Moderation in all things," and "Too much of a good thing can kill you"? Don't overfeed, overstarve, overstress, overexercise, overtan, or over-anything your body. Don't ingest or inhale things that are going to stress out your systems.

Oh, and don't be overly bound by all the don'ts in your life! Eat some sweets—they do add to the sweetness of life. (Like most women, I love chocolate and relish recent findings that suggest it is actually good for you.)

Eat some foods you enjoy that may not be on the health-food list but can be worked into balance with plenty of other nutritious foods. Get some sunshine—it will brighten your perspective and contribute vitamin D to your body. Get some exercise. Work hard and rest well.

Balance is key. This is wisdom of old. Certainly, competitive athletes must exercise harder than most of us, and physical laborers must push their bodies. Yet even they will benefit mentally and physically if they can find a rhythm of hard work and rest.

I am not against working hard. I believe our bodies were created for it. But we function more peacefully when we balance work with rest. We must stop feeling guilty about resting, stop seeing it as a luxury, and start recognizing that it is necessary for a more peaceful life and a sense of well-being. Too much rest, on the other hand, is out of balance and not good for you, either.

Be balanced in eating, exercising, and resting. It will bring peace to your body.

Here are some things I do to bring peace and gentleness to my body.

I walk. Walking is extremely beneficial to our bodies. It strengthens muscles, bones, and our cardiovascular systems. It also relieves stress and brings peace of mind. And it's easy and enjoyable. Best of all, it's something I'll actually do. I love the European saying "Why ride when you can walk?" I think all of us would feel a lot better if we walked more.

I build strength. We can do this in a number of ways without leaving the comforts of home, but I go to a women's fitness center (it's less intimidating than a general fitness center!) for thirty minutes three times a week to keep my muscles toned and to maintain my posture. This promotes overall health and good posture, which makes us look slimmer. It's fun and not too time consuming.

I get regular massages. I know this is a stretch for some people. It's taken me years to justify it, but massage definitely brings peace to your body. It's great for circulation and helps rid your body of toxins, stress, and tension. I consider this an investment in my overall health. Of course, it can be expensive, and at times I've had to strike it from our budget because it looked too much like a luxury. But even having family members massage each other's hands and feet is beneficial. Touch goes a long way toward calming our bodies, healing them, and promoting a sense of well-being. I think singles and the elderly might need this most of all.

I take time out for quiet. I have some time to myself early in the morning over coffee (yes, I do indulge!). I look forward to this time, so it is not a discipline but a treat. With my busy household and responsibilities, this is the only time that is quiet enough for me to think. I read the Bible and pray. I ponder big ideas and think through smaller ones, like how I am going to get a certain project done or answer someone who sent me an e-mail the day before. I think about how I can be a better wife, a better mom, a better friend. Since I do a lot of public speaking, I think about what I am going to say. Usually the ideas come to me in this time, and I formulate my outlines during these early moments in my day. We all need time to think, to organize, to ponder. It will help us be better, more thoughtful people.

I eat yogurt. It calms the digestive system (if you are not lactose intolerant).

I enjoy some time outdoors. Fresh air does wonders for lifting my countenance and giving me a brighter perspective—even if it involves rain or wind blowing in my face. It gently refreshes me.

These are a few of my systems for bringing peace to my body. None of these are too costly or time consuming, except massage, but you can find a way around that. Actually, they are all pretty simple.

Yet too often we avoid such methods because we can't justify their sharing equal value with our work. So we work on and stress out and become increasingly overweight or underweight and unhealthy and then need forced rest. Why not build a few patterns into our lifestyles now that promote peace rather than stress? They don't have to be complicated. Actually, the simpler they are, the better the odds that you'll do them. They'll also help you enjoy your life more every day.

TAKE TIME FOR BEAUTY

Beauty is a gift we give to others. Taking time for beauty is a way to show our loved ones we value them. Think about it. Does it show your husband or your children you value them when you look like a slob around the house? I don't mean that you have to have your makeup on at all times, but you should at least look as if you take care of yourself. Your family should be proud to be seen with you even if you're camping and you're not wearing makeup and your hair is pulled back in a ponytail. You can look beautiful even then, simply because you take care of yourself in a reasonable way.

Each of us has to develop comfortable methods and habits to help us look our best. Again, they don't have to be elaborate—remember, focusing too much on ourselves actually works against us (no matter how good we think we look). Our systems should be simple—the kind we'll do and keep on doing.

Here are a few of mine:

Take five. I recite this little phrase in my mind every night before bed and every morning when I first wake up. I developed it when my children were little. I would be so exhausted at night that I could hardly see my way to bed in order to collapse. My older sister had told me that every night I failed to take off my makeup before bed aged my face by seven days. So I would tell myself, "Gayle, just take five." This meant just take five minutes to brush my teeth, wash my face, moisturize it, brush my hair, and dress for bed. This I could do—just five minutes, and I would feel and look better. (This also works wonders for your marriage!)

Then in the morning I would do the same thing. Take five. Brush my teeth, wash and moisturize my face, and brush my hair. Showering, blow-drying my hair, and putting on makeup take a little more time, and I work these into my morning schedule after quiet time and exercise. But every morning I take five, even when camping.

Set aside time once a week for pampering. Pampering sounds like a luxury, but really it is a necessity to keep your body and face looking as though you care about yourself. This is the time to care for hands and feet, fingernails and toenails, to shave your legs, exfoliate, and use a facial mask. This takes about an hour, which is a small investment toward looking your best and feeling more confident about yourself. Doing this regularly keeps me from needing professional facials, manicures, and pedicures. (It always encourages me, how-ever, when women ask me where I've gone to have these done.)

Be reasonable with your diet. This is where the Jerusalem Diet helps me. I like foods that are good for me, and most of my diet consists of these foods. But I also love sweets, particularly chocolate, as I mentioned earlier, and ice cream. I believe these foods contribute to my sense of well-being as long as I don't overdo it. I can get grouchy when I haven't eaten them in a while, which affects the well-being of those around me.

Even so, these indulgences that oversupply me with fat can affect my weight. So when my weight starts to climb, I take a day or two, sometimes three, and just eat fruits, vegetables, nuts, and seeds. This is an easy discipline for me, because I feel so good when I do it—and I never feel hungry. I even feel some of the same healthy effects on my body that I get from fasting—without the hunger and discomfort. It's a no-lose situation (except for the pounds). I feel better, and my weight is under control.

Exercise. I've already discussed the value of exercise in bringing peace to our bodies. Of course, exercise also helps us look better. Alternating walking with strength building, I exercise thirty to forty-five minutes, five to six times a week. On my Fat Days, I exercise fifteen minutes more.

These four beauty systems are simple. They take a little time and effort but produce wonderful benefits as they help me look and feel better for myself and my loved ones.

DON'T QUIT

We should see our lives as a process that begins at conception and continues until we die. We are always learning, growing, changing, and—I hope—improving all the way through life. I think we should view our failures in diet and exercise as part of the process—not a series of personal disasters but a continuation of our process to improve ourselves.

My exhortation to you is to keep going. Don't ever give up. You might suffer a few setbacks that last a day, a week, or even a year or two. But don't tell yourself you have to start over. Instead, reevaluate, come up with a plan, and keep going.

As you adopt this perspective, you begin to see that you can take care of yourself every day—exercise some, eat better, take five—without requiring a major overhaul. If you don't do well one day, get up the next morning, weigh yourself, take five, exercise, eat fruits, vegetables, nuts, and seeds, if necessary, and have a great day.

Good days begin to add up over time, and you will grow healthier and probably improve your appearance and sense of well-being. Occasionally you may even throw in a more intensive diet or exercise program, but I'd advise that you always return to this basic system. You will continue to receive the benefits throughout your life. *Just don't quit.*

I've been exercising regularly in some fashion since high school. I've missed some days, even weeks here and there, but I've always seen this as a way of life, so I just keep going. I don't have any high athletic aspirations. I just exercise because it is good for me. I've found the greatest benefits have come not in my short-term goals but rather in the long term of just doing it week after week.

If you haven't exercised in a while, get up tomorrow morning, find the exercise you enjoy and your doctor approves, and pick up where you last left off.

SMILE

My final tip to you is to smile.

When I was a young girl, I read that the best way to start your day is to smile. So I wrote the letters S M I L E on a piece of paper and taped it to the ceiling above my bed. Even then, I felt a little awkward forcing my mouth into a smile first thing in the morning. Yet, as my mouth slowly broadened into a smile, I felt my perspective brighten. I lay there on my bed during those first few moments of the morning just feeling happy about the day ahead. I still do this from time to time (minus the paper on the ceiling), and it still works.

I've also learned that if I am caught with no makeup on or if I'm having a bad hair or body day, smiling helps get me through and keeps me looking good in the eyes of others.

Regardless of our size, shape, or health condition, we can all utilize this greatest beauty secret of all—kindness. The world longs for kindhearted women and always finds them beautiful. Just look at the world's-most-admired-women lists from a few years back: Mother Teresa and Princess Diana led the list because of their acts of kindness. Was Princess Diana ever more beautiful than when she was looking into the face of her boys and smiling? I don't think so. Those pictures take my breath away. And who doesn't look at the deeply wrinkled face of Mother Teresa and see her tremendous beauty?

Being kinder to yourself and thoughtful toward others—that's the subject of my chapter, but it's also part of Ted's motivation for writing this book. We don't want you to be miserable all your life. We all have so much to be grateful for. Life is wonderful. Enjoy yours as much as possible, and help others to do the same.

When my husband asked me to write this chapter, it reminded me of how fortunate I am. You see, my husband thinks I am beautiful. He thinks that I am the ideal weight for me and that I am in great shape. I, on the other hand, am aware of how many pounds over my ideal weight I am (according to most of the current charts) and of the evidence that still exists around my middle that I've given birth to five children. Yet over time I've learned to accept my body and to work with it peaceably and with joy—and that is my favorite beauty secret. At least, it has worked in the eyes of my husband and children—the people I love and care about most.

CHAPTER 13

Break Addictions

My wife likes to begin her day with a cup of coffee. There are people in our offices who keep a pot brewing all day long, and I'm sure some of the folks on my staff have bought stock in Starbucks. At least, they should have, because they seem to be single-handedly keeping the company profitable.

I'm fortunate not to like the taste of coffee. But by now you know I have little room to brag. Mountain Dew is the nectar of the gods, as far as I'm concerned, and in addition to caffeine it has enough sugar to turn my stomach into a cotton candy machine.

But then I'm not addicted. I love the stuff, but I don't get headaches when I don't drink it. I don't get the shakes or have any kind of withdrawal symptoms. Well, my heart does ache a little, but it's more like puppy-love heartache.

Actually, I'm not sure if I've ever been addicted to anything the way people are addicted to coffee. I have deep cravings, but if I don't get what I want, my body doesn't react in any perceivable way. I can't think of a day I spent writhing in pain because I didn't get my fix of Jelly Bellies, and I've never seriously considered psychological treatment for my boundless affection for Mountain Dew.

If you're going to do the Jerusalem Diet well, you should try to break whatever addictions you have. Caffeine may not be the demon from hell that some people make it out to be—according to Dr. Walter Willett, coffee has the advantage of fighting kidney stones and gallstones[1]—but you don't want to be so addicted that you can't function without a daily fix. If skipping coffee in the morning means you'll be bedridden all day, writhing in migraine-like agony, you may have a problem.

Get this: after the most recent long-term study of caffeine use at Johns Hopkins School of Medicine, the researchers recommended that caffeine addiction be included in the next version of the *Diagnostic and Statistical Manual of Mental Disorders,* the guidebook for mental-health professionals. The Johns Hopkins researchers found that drinking as little as one cup of coffee per day—when eliminated—can cause withdrawal symptoms ranging from mild headaches to much worse problems, including depression, inability to focus, and flulike symptoms.[2]

Now, even though they think of caffeine withdrawal as a real disorder because the symptoms are so pronounced, the researchers hesitate to make a big deal out of caffeine addiction. The withdrawals don't last long (a few days at most), and all coffee and tea users can quit if they choose to.

As with everything in the Jerusalem Diet, I don't want you to beat yourself up about this. Caffeine won't kill you; you just don't want to be addicted to anything. You want to be more flexible than that. You want to be able to go without something if you need to or just want to. So as you read this, if the thought of going without coffee—or any one thing—is making you consider driving over my dog, then go ahead and admit you have a problem. You can get over the addiction—just stop drinking it one day when you don't need to function at your highest level. Take an ibuprofen to get through the withdrawal if you need to. After you're past the tough part, you can return to drinking caffeine in moderation and with self-control.

Let me say something about addictions in general, whether the addiction be to cigarettes, alcohol, coffee, tea, sugar, or anything else. You don't absolutely need any of those things, and you'd be better off if you could enjoy them on different terms (except cigarettes and alcohol). Don't be a slave to anything. Be free. Don't let any substance determine how you live your day. Coffee culture is wonderful—the smell of it, cool coffeehouses, great conversations—but you're not able to appreciate it if you're mainlining the stuff every day. Desserts are fantastic, but you aren't really enjoying them if you're always obsessing about the amount of time between sweets.

The problem of addictions has to do with more than what you put into your body. As a pastor, I see people who are addicted to all kinds of things, and their lives would be so much better if they could be free. People get addicted to cars, BlackBerries (the PDAs, not the fruit), video games, pornography, bad relationships, laziness, television shows, and more. Contemporary culture has done a great job of giving us more and more things to be addicted to, so people with addictive tendencies can pretty well wrap up their lives in numerous habits.

I just want to say thank you for sharing the Jerusalem Diet. I am the average American—thirty to forty pounds overweight. I feel so blessed that I finally found something that is simple and that I can fit into my lifestyle.

I struggled during my teenage years with anorexia and bulimia, and since then I've been up and down on fad diets. I did them until I was exhausted and sad. For once I am seeing success. I have lost twenty pounds and have twenty more to go—halfway there! I feel strong and confident.

Thank you,

Kim

A friend of mine says that addictions are one of the central problems in his life. He says he has an addictive personality—not that people get addicted to him, but that he gets addicted to everything. He doesn't struggle with the usual suspects—coffee, cigarettes, alcohol, or anything so obvious—but things that are more deceptively addicting, like compulsively listening to sports radio and NPR or talking on the phone in any potential moment of silence. A couple of years ago he was addicted to newspapers. Every morning he would read the local paper, the *New York Times*, the *Wall Street Journal*, the *Economist*, and *USA Today*. If he skipped one, it would nag at him all day long.

This doesn't sound like a big deal, but this guy couldn't (or wouldn't) function without his daily newspaper routine. As silly as it sounds, his paper-reading habit was messing with his life, and he had to pull himself away so that reading the daily news could have its proper place.

That's the best argument for breaking whatever addictions you have in your life—keeping everything in its proper place. Some addictions—cigarettes, illegal drugs, pornography—are purely detrimental and shouldn't have any place in your life. But some addictions are less innocuous and perhaps harder to recognize. Either way, addictions need to be uprooted so you can be free.

I want you to enjoy your life. I want you to be free.

CHAPTER 14

Use Failure to Your Advantage

My wife and I went to Hawaii this year. Gayle did great on the trip. She ordered healthy foods at the restaurants, munched on the fancy fruits that were available all day long, and exercised in the warm weather. For breakfast, she had papaya and strawberries. She loved the fresh tomato and mozzarella cheese slices with basil for lunch. For dinner she ate fish and vegetables. She was incredible. She took long walks on the beach and did calisthenics in the room.

It's no wonder she weighs the same as she did before we got married, even after having five children. While on vacation, she was more health conscious than normal, if that's possible.

But not me. I got fat.

I ate heavy breakfasts, which I don't normally do. I had nut-and-banana pancakes, oatmeal, omelets, waffles, and fruit. I enjoyed crunchy grilled french toast, huevos rancheros, breakfast burritos, and eggs Benedict. These foods, complete with English muffins, Canadian bacon, and cheese, were wonderful. For lunch I had whatever was nearby, no matter how fattening. Then I would have big dinners. I would go to bed so full that I felt like I couldn't roll over.

Ever been there?

Probably not. I'm the worst.

Because my big breakfasts made me sleepy, instead of joining Gayle for laps in the pool, I took a quick nap. By the time I joined her, she had exercised for a good hour and was relaxing with a thick book. The pool water looked nice, but I wanted to lie next to my wife and listen to the sounds of the pool or the surf. I hopped in the water long enough to feel cool and refreshed (much needed after my nap!), then grabbed some magazines or a book and sat back in the sun with her, only to fall asleep while she read. Then we went to a long, leisurely lunch. We'd walk around a bit, then I'd want another nap. Then snacks. At long last we'd dress up and go out for a great evening meal with several courses and delicious desserts.

It was a fantastic vacation. I came home several pounds overweight, but I enjoyed gaining every single one of those pounds. I used to do it every vacation. During my normal business trips, which happen almost every week, it's no problem to stay on the Jerusalem Diet. At times I enjoy using hotel gyms and eating healthy food in restaurants. But on vacation, sometimes I go limp. The more my trajectory changes toward health, the less it happens, but it still happens. The walls of self-control come tumbling down, and I give in to my aching desires to eat, sleep, and eat some more.

Because the Jerusalem Diet is such a consistent, easy lifestyle, when I come home a few pounds above my ideal weight, I start my first day home at my current weight and use a calendar to lower my weekly target weight by one pound a week. With this system I don't have to announce my failure, I don't have to go on a binge diet, and I don't have to writhe in guilt because of my foolish excesses. Instead, I fix it.

Whatever weight I gain while away from home—whether one pound or ten—will come off eventually, even if I have to work a little harder than in years past. As I've said before, for most people it's easier to gain weight than to lose it. And it's easier to lose weight the younger you are. So as you go through the years, it's best to get to your ideal weight and stay there.

But never be discouraged if you get off your plan for any reason (vacation, tragedy in the family). Just start again from wherever you are.

Healthy, Not Skinny

This might be a good place to mention the problem with ideal weights. The ideal weight on a chart is often, in my opinion, too slender for people. The reason our bodies store additional weight as we get older is so we'll have a reserve of stored energy should we get sick. I've seen older men and women who look terrible at their ideal weight. In my nonprofessional opinion, they were so skinny that it looked as if they would die if they got sick. They had no reserve.

I think it's okay for us to achieve our ideal weight, then evaluate if it is too thin for us. Once we reach our ideal weight, we all need to do some form of resistance training to build muscle, but even with that, you might look too skinny. If so, my guess is that you'll look and feel great somewhere between your official ideal weight and about ten pounds over.

At five pounds over, you'll look stunning at the pool. At your ideal weight, you may look fabulous at the pool, but in your clothes you may appear skinny. This is totally subjective, but it's a Haggard guideline you might want to follow. I've found that people enjoy some flexibility in working with their ideal weight.

Your goal is not to look anorexic or even like a supermodel (which is often the same thing). You just want to look and be as healthy as you can.

This is why I'm not alarmed if I go on vacation and have a wonderful time relaxing and, in the midst of it, plunge into Slurpees, steaks, and sandwiches. These times of real, prolonged relaxation are rare for me, and it's worth gaining a little bit so that my body and mind can really rest.

NEW THINKING ABOUT SUCCESS AND FAILURE

If you've struggled with your weight for a long time, you probably need to start thinking differently about success and failure. It's the direction your life is taking—the overall trajectory—that is important. Where you are today is not as important as the direction you are headed toward tomorrow. No doubt, we want to avoid major failures—things that would cost us our lives, our relationships, our careers—but in some areas, we also want to avoid major successes.

Sounds strange, right? Well, I could have succeeded at dieting on my vacation, but I would have missed a wonderful time of needed relaxation.

Think about people who become rich very quickly, leaving their families in the dust as they pursue dollar after dollar. Think about people who achieve major fame. Our culture celebrates them for a little while, but eventually we hear about their dark underbelly, because in their sprint toward success, they left some important things behind.

These sprints toward success and plunges into failure are exactly what we want to avoid. We will experience both failure and success in our lives, but we need to manage them carefully. The best-lived life includes little failures that provide a chance for correction and a series of little successes that build into the one great success of a good life.

Let's say you are experiencing one of those little failures. You are fat. You have gone back to your old way of living. What should you do?

Start over tomorrow morning. Just the thought that you are going to do something proactive, yet easy, tomorrow should make the rest of today hopeful. Then, in the morning, weigh yourself and start the plan. That means tomorrow you will be at your target weight for the week, but you can't be foolish. This first week will stop the growth of the bulge and the flab and start your body in the other direction.

Again, I encourage people to read all the diet, exercise, and nutrition books they like and do them as long as they can, even if they are also doing the Jerusalem Diet. Why? Because every improvement in what you eat should fit into the overall plan of moving your weight toward your ideal weight and keeping it there. The Jerusalem Diet is the umbrella plan that just about any other plan will fit under.

The major difference: on this plan you emphasize real food but don't exclude everything. Shop in the produce department. Eat and drink authentic food. Enjoy the wiggle room to be as human as you would like, within reason.

So some days you'll be on fruits, vegetables, nuts, seeds, water, and exercise. On other days you can do what I often do when I'm on target. I eat fruits, vegetables, nuts, and seeds, drink water throughout the day, enjoy some exercise, and have whatever I want at dinner, ensuring that I'm finished by 7:00 p.m. Then I enjoy yogurt, cottage cheese with fruit, or a bowl of cereal just before bed. Heaven!

Let's say you like the way I use the diet, but some days you don't exercise. Fine. If you have an eating plan like the one I just outlined and exercise moderately three times a week, you'll never be heavy again.

But remember: failure on this plan is no ticket to despair. Have an overall idea of what is good and what is not.

If you go to the movies or are cooking around the campfire, you can have some popcorn and a Coke or a roasted marshmallow or a hot dog. You'll handle it just fine. It won't throw you off, and you won't have a Fat Day tomorrow because of it. Why? Because you are into the lifestyle, and your body is not fighting you; it's not feeling abused by you. Instead, it is working with you and rejoicing in the real food you are also giving it.

You only have to be strict on the plan if you are over your target. And only for one day. Weigh yourself daily and live accordingly.

Failure is not the end of the world. Just start again tomorrow. Some days your life is just going to be too busy to hit the gym or jog around the neighborhood. That's okay. Over the course of the next few years, it'd be best if you exercised more and more, and that's what you should shoot for. But little slip-ups along the way are okay.

Some days you'll be a pound or two over your target weight because you went on a late Krispy Kreme binge the night before. But those three leftover doughnuts in the refrigerator are too tempting to withstand, and you give in again. It's okay. If you do that, rather than let the total day be a failure, spend the rest of the day recovering and eating real food. You may be over your target again tomorrow, and if so, it gives you another opportunity to have a little success.

As a Christian pastor, I have an idea about failure, which I can sum up pretty easily: God loves us. He cares about us and wants us to do well. When we fail, he wants us to be open to correction, and he also wants us to rebound. He wants us to learn, to improve, to get better as we learn through trial and error. So when we fail, we need to realize that we're not trapped by that failure. We're free to try again and again. We are on the road to victory, and there are going to be speed bumps along the way.

Failure is not devastating for me. Why? We're talking about a one-pound goal, not thirty or fifty pounds. I'm never *that* far off.

The world of Haggard is a wonderful place.

CHAPTER 15

Shop Like You Mean It

Dieting decisions get made in the aisles of a grocery store. What you put in your basket, you'll put in your fridge and pantry. What you put in your fridge and pantry, you'll put in your body. So start by being careful about what goes in that basket.

I like to use my instincts to shop. Lots of diet guides say never shop when you are hungry. I don't think so. I'm *always* hungry when I shop.

And I always start my shopping in the produce department.

A lot of grocers put the produce near the front door so you have to walk through and see all those beautiful colors and smell all those amazing smells. It's very smart of them, and it works on me every time. I load the cart with apples (I like Gala and Red Delicious), grapefruit, bananas (a little green so they'll ripen and be good for several days), kiwis, lemons and limes, avocados, tomatoes, and on and on. The produce section often has all the things you need for good salads, including nuts and seeds. I love buying everything we need for several days of great salads. Mmmm. There's nothing like romaine lettuce with chunks of red apple, walnuts, and raisins.

I love to load a salad with peppers, too. But why are green peppers so much more affordable than red, orange, and yellow peppers? I love them all, and when we can afford it, we splurge on all those tasty peppers. I especially love them sautéed with onion and mixed with my scrambled eggs.

But anyway, back at the store, picking up broccoli and asparagus, cucumbers and carrots. Sometimes as I go through the produce section and the rest of the aisles, I use a list, but other times we've not planned specific meals, so we just buy whatever looks good. Or whatever is on sale.

Do we stop at the deli counter? Well, this is a tough choice for some people. The cheeses are usually great, but some nutritionists tell you to stay away from processed meats, which includes pretty much all the great sandwich meat behind the counter. Unless you have a specific health reason to avoid these meats altogether, I think you can carefully choose some deli meats that are not processed very heavily. Sandwich meat can be expensive, though, and frankly, I think salads make better lunches.

When health-food stores first became popular in Colorado Springs, I admit I was a little freaked out by them. It seemed to me that the people in those stores looked a little sickly—a little too thin, a little peaked. And the stores smelled funny, like a combination of a produce farm and a massage-therapy office.

But I figured out that there's some pretty amazing stuff in those places, and shopping in them can be a heavenly experience. On a good day they will give you dinner as you shop, that is, if you take advantage of all the samples. The cheese section makes you feel like you're in Paris, and the coffee aisle is like a trip to Seattle—or so my wife says. Only the best ice creams are available, alongside frozen meals that make the TV dinners of old look like mess-hall leftovers. The best organic stores feature delicatessens with a full team of chefs putting together organic lasagnas, veggie burgers, chicken wraps, and sushi plates. Oh, it's incredible! With all these choices I would still choose organic pizza.

Yes, it gets pretty pricey. The great thing about the free-market system, however, is that as people patronize these places, they are becoming more affordable. And as organic foods become more popular, the regular grocery chains will feature an ever-growing stock with competitive prices.

Still, for now, organic food, whether bought from an organic food outlet or a regular grocery store, can be expensive. Don't break the bank on organic produce. If you can afford only the conventionally grown produce at the regular grocery chain, eat it. It contains nutrients that are good for you. Our bodies are beautifully and wonderfully made. It's amazing how complex our bodies are and how capable they are of processing most of the foods we eat.

The main thing to remember is to eat real food. The more real the food is, the better it is for you. Organic food is better than food saturated in pesticides.

I am fifty years old and have been a lifelong athlete—long-distance runner and squash, tennis, and racquetball player. During college I lived on Heartbreak Hill in Boston and ran part of the Boston Marathon course daily. I maintained a weight of 172 pounds from my freshman year until just a few years ago.

At age forty-seven I had to stop running due to knee problems. I quickly gained twenty pounds, despite regular treadmill and biking time. For three years I wrestled with the weight. I tried various diets, and everything failed miserably. My weight stayed stubbornly above 190 pounds.

As soon as I heard you speak on the Jerusalem Diet, I started it. I had immediate and steady progress, and as of this morning, I weigh 180 pounds. I feel great. It has been painless. I have eaten well, and I've not had to turn into an ascetic.

I'm shooting for an ideal weight of a lean, mean 178 pounds. I expect to be there in two more weeks, and best of all, I'm confident that I'll maintain that weight. Thanks for passing on this great tool!

Scott

Natural food is better than highly processed food. Whole grains are better than grains that have been broken down. Brown rice is better than white rice. A peanut is better than a Nutter Butter. Water and juice are better than soda.

This is obvious, right? But it's hard to apply, because those Nutter Butters are oh so good. So eat those, too, but not in direct proportion to the number of peanuts you eat.

SHOPPING ON A BUDGET

Grocery bills can ruin a budget. It's tough to rein in food spending, and as you add kids to your family, it gets even harder. Dieters should be able to do better at this than nondieters, because being careful about what you put in your basket means there shouldn't be any surprises at the checkout. And though some diet foods are expensive, you can buy plenty of regular foods that are healthy for you and aren't subject to markups because some famous dieting guru endorsed them.

Don't fall into the trap of believing that you have to spend lots of money to eat healthy food. You can do a protein-heavy, carb-light diet for very little money. Just about every grocer has some meat on sale every weekend, and you can cook the meat with whatever herbs, spices, or oils you have on hand and serve it with a salad.

You're getting protein, you're getting vegetables and all their nutrients, you're avoiding excess overprocessed carbs, and you're saving money. You can splurge on the rosemary and olive focaccia another time.

CHAPTER 16

Drink Your Fruits and Vegetables

Not long ago Gayle and I went to a basketball game, and on our way home we stopped and ate Krispy Kreme doughnuts. They were delightful, and we felt fine. The next morning we thought we might pay for our doughnut sins, but when we weighed ourselves, we were both under our target weight for the day. Score! Got away with one!

But because I had been a little bad the night before, I wanted to be extra healthy at breakfast. Instead of pouring a bowl of Honey Nut Cheerios, I juiced two tomatoes and drank those.

It's not unusual for me to do that. Sometimes I want to sit down and have breakfast, but most mornings I'm on my way out the door shortly after I get out of bed. If my weight is on target or under and if I have time, I'll have an egg on toast with cheese and some fresh orange juice. But more often, whether I have ten minutes or an hour for breakfast, I fire up the blender or the juicer. I love drinking tomatoes because they're a superfood with a host of nutrients that both give me immediate energy and promote long-term health (more on this later). But I'll drink whatever fruits or vegetables we have lying around the counter or stored in the crisper and freezer. Sometimes I'll cut up a banana, pour in orange juice, add frozen blueberries, and turn on the juicer. Sometimes I'll just juice a whole cucumber.

I've mentioned the blender and the juicer before. The difference between the two is that while the juicer extracts the juice, it discards the pulp and seeds, but the blender mixes it all together. The blender gives you more nutrients because it uses all of the produce.

Sometimes I love the juicer, because the juice tastes so refreshing, and it feels as if all the good nutrients are going straight into my cells. But when I use it, I know I'm not getting the skin, which is often the most nutrient-rich part of the fruit or vegetable. Juicing doesn't give you enough fiber, which is a major benefit to eating fruits and vegetables.

Blenders are great! You can toss in two tomatoes with a cup of water and know that you are drinking the whole tomato. You can do that with all kinds of things. In the summertime you can take apples and strawberries and oranges and blend them all together, and it's fabulous. You get every single good thing that those foods have to offer.

As you do things like that, your body changes its orientation. Soon it switches from craving a Big Mac to craving a blended tomato. At least, that's what happened to me.

There is one significant caveat to my fondness for the blender and juicer. They are great for fast breakfasts and postexercise refreshments. But in general, I'd say that if you want strawberries, eat strawberries. You can drink ten strawberries in three seconds by using a blender, but that may put food into your system too fast. Chewing is good for you—it burns calories! And chewing jump-starts your digestive system.

I learned about the benefits of a blender from people who were healthy but a little overweight. I was hesitant because of that. After getting my own blender and realizing that it was so easy to make strawberry slushes and mix fruits and vegetables, I saw how addicting it could be. And it dawned on me: this is good, but it's still not as good as eating whole fruits and vegetables.

In the orchard we pick fruits, not fruit juice.

In the garden we harvest vegetables in a certain form, not as a liquid.

When I have time, I eat fruits and vegetables. But there is nothing as energizing and refreshing as using the juicer or blender to get a refreshing, nutrition-packed drink.

In recent years juice and smoothie bars have been the rage, partly because they sell "boosts" that you can add to your drink for a few more cents (by "a few more" they mean at least fifty). Those drinks are very tasty, but if you're interested in losing weight, you should stay away from them. There are tons of calories in many of those drinks, especially ones made with sherbet or yogurt. And at the end of the day, calories do count.

But juicing and blending are good for you as long as you don't overdo it. I've already mentioned how the various phytochemicals found in vegetables and fruits can protect against cancer and heart disease. In particular, tomato juice contains lycopene, a phytochemical that prevents prostate cancer. In one study, people who drank six ounces of tomato juice a day experienced a 43 percent increase of lycopene levels in their blood in addition to increases in other carotenoid substances. In my mind, this is enough reason to make drinking fruits and vegetables a regular habit in addition to eating them with meals. Here is the bottom line: sure, you can take pills, eat junk, exercise a little, and see how you come out. But it's so easy to use the Jerusalem Diet method to get the food the way you were designed to get it.

Many people take their fruits and vegetables in pill form. That's certainly better than not getting fruits and vegetables at all. And many of us take vitamins in megadoses, thinking it will make us healthy. I know some people have experienced health gains with such vitamin use, but my guess is that, in the future, researchers will determine that when we get things out of balance, we create problems we never imagined. All of us appreciate vitamins C and E and many other "miracle" vitamins, but getting C and E in their natural, balanced form will do more for us than taking them in megadoses.

So eat fruits and vegetables. If you can't eat them, drink them. If you can't drink them, take them as a pill. But remember, we're on a continuum from worst (no fruits and vegetables at all), to pills and drinks, to the real thing in the form God provided.

Doctors are concerned that people who drink fruit juices don't necessarily eat less. This can be a problem, so you'll need to be careful not to drink so much that you mess with your weight.

Also, if you get into the habit of drinking fruits and vegetables, don't let it take the place of drinking regular water. Many people are dehydrated because they don't get enough water but instead fill themselves with sodas. As good as sodas taste, they have absolutely zero nutritional value.[1]

I said it earlier, but let me say it again: water makes your body work. It's the main ingredient of all the fluids in your body, from your blood to your digestive juices. Water will help your body deal better with food, from good digestion to proper waste elimination. Think about all the mucus that's inside your eyes and nasal glands—all that goo you may have seen when someone's body is sliced open in surgery on television. That mucus is a necessary lubricant to keep your body machine functioning, and you need to drink water to keep the mucus adequate and effective.

Okay, it's obvious by now that I'm no expert, but I believe that many people who are sick are actually thirsty. I also believe that often when people get foggy and can't think or remember, they are thirsty. Their brains need more water. Your body needs water to function properly even if you are not very active. Your lungs like humid air, so the body uses three to four cups of water per day on breathing alone!

Drink a big glass of water when you get up in the morning and another

I attended your talk not because I'm overweight but because I'm middle-aged, and during the last ten years my metabolism has slowed down. Before that I was always very thin—about 120 pounds—but able to eat like two men. I love food, I love to cook, and I love to serve people by making fantastic, complicated meals.

But as I've come into my forties, I've begun to struggle, because my food no longer just passes on by; it thinks I should wear it. Some time ago my fasting times started to have mixed motives between seeking God and trying to lose weight rapidly. I decided to go to your talk because I wondered if I was on the verge of becoming bulimic.

I was so happy to hear you say that you really love to eat. I loved the idea of not having to have self-control every single day but only on days when I'm over my target weight. And the idea of eating only fruits, vegetables, nuts, and seeds some days also sounded very entertaining to me since I enjoy just about any kind of food a person can put in front of me, and there's plenty of room for variety in that list.

At first while doing the Jerusalem Diet, I cheated a lot, because I was so happy I didn't have to be legalistic! But I've discovered that a handful of nuts and seeds in the morning fills me up for hours. The longer I do it, the less I add extras to the vegetables I eat. I'm finally experiencing the self-control I've been without my whole life.

I talk about the diet to people everywhere I go: in the YMCA and in stores, to anyone, anywhere, whether I know them or not. It's easy. People like to hear good news.

Thank you,

Pam

when you go to bed at night. On your Fat Days, drink more water. It will help you drop weight. Have a full glass of something with every meal and some water between meals.[2] Don't necessarily wait until you're thirsty—thirst doesn't always develop immediately when the body needs fluid. Beat thirst to the punch by staying hydrated all day, first with water, then with other liquids at your discretion.

Is it possible to drink too much water? I think it is.

Several years ago I had major voice problems, and as you might know, voice problems can result from the vocal folds not being adequately hydrated. Consequently, my doctor told me to sip water throughout the day and to drink a big glass of water in the morning and at night before bed. He emphasized that even though I might need to get up and go to the bathroom in the middle of the night, the water working through my system to refresh and cleanse it was worth it.

I overdid it at the beginning, drinking voraciously whenever I was thirsty. As a result, I didn't feel good. My doctor laughed. He said that, as a rule of thumb, I needed to monitor the hydration of my body by the color of my urine. I should try to pee pale. In other words, if my urine is yellow or any bright color or has an odor, then I need more water. If it is clear, I am too hydrated and should back off. If it is pale, that's perfect. This varies some, depending on vitamins and minerals being filtered through the body. So dark pee is not always a bad sign, but in general, peeing pale is a good rule.

I know this method is easier for men than for women, but it's helpful for all. Any of us can check throughout the day to ensure that our hydration is sufficient and that our bodies are working well.

So drink up—fruits and vegetables in moderation and lots of water!

CHAPTER 17

Eat Early and Get a Good Night's Rest

I love to sleep. I'm one of the few people in the world who is disappointed that we only sleep one-third of our lives away. I love the feel of the sheets. I love falling asleep. I love waking up from time to time in the middle of the night to go to the bathroom and read, pray, and just think. Why? Because I so enjoy going back to sleep.

I also like snoozing—going back to bed in the morning to get a little more sleep. I did that this morning. I woke up at 5:30, answered *sixty-five* e-mails, and went back to sleep. It was great, because I knew I didn't have appointments today, no flights to catch, no activities to rush my children to. I had the chance to stay in bed as long as I wanted. So I woke up late, grabbed my laptop, and began to write while still in bed. It was great.

Many in the world of fitness underestimate sleep. Or at least they under-emphasize it. If we would get proper sleep, our temperaments, spiritual lives, and health would be better. In the past I've had a series of Fat Days that I wasn't able to get a handle on, and then, with two or three good nights of sleep in a row, I found myself feeling better and found that my weight had adjusted again.

Sleep is a gift from God to reset our bodies, to file information we've learned, to give our minds and bodies an opportunity to reorganize and strengthen. Sleep brings a pleasing order.

Unless, of course, we've overeaten just before going to bed.

I've already spoken about not eating anything significant after 7:00 p.m. I think in my process of learning the Jerusalem Diet, this was the biggest hurdle for me. I used to like going to bed with a full stomach. As a kid and as a young man, I would go to sleep easier on a full stomach. But I'm convinced this habit was the number one reason I started to get fat.

Sure, I needed more real food, and I needed a plan to get down to my ideal weight, and I needed a system of exercise. But even as I began to achieve those things, if I ate late at night, my sleep wouldn't be as peaceful. It was as if I could actually feel the late-night meal going straight to my fat cells and causing them to grow.

Late-night eating doesn't do us any good. These days I hate going to bed with a full stomach. I feel like a slob. I feel like a loser. I feel as if I'm shortening my life and overworking all my systems by eating late. So I try not to eat too late and instead drink a glass of water before bed and maybe have yogurt or a bowl of cereal. I don't want to be hungry, but I also don't want to be full.

My job requirements are such that sometimes I go several days on little sleep, and I'm usually okay during those stretches. But I'm okay only because I know that I'm merely postponing one of the best experiences this side of heaven: deep, deep sleep. When my long work nights are over, I love recuperating. I love climbing into bed, finding that perfect position, and sleeping soundly and peacefully.

When I eat healthy, I sleep healthy. There is a direct correlation between the way that I eat and the way that I sleep. It is part of the continuum of good health. In general, if I'm being careful about what goes into my body, I'm being careful about how I rest. So, for me, this is another reason to weigh myself first thing in the morning and be deliberate about what I put in my mouth all day. I know if I am careful to do that, I'll also rest better.

EATING AFFECTS SLEEPING, AND SLEEPING AFFECTS EATING

Let me give you a couple of scientific explanations for why sleeping well and eating well go hand in hand. Last fall a CBS News report based on an article in the *Journal of Clinical Endocrinology and Metabolism* suggested that there is a link between obesity and sleep deprivation. The article explained that all of

I hate dieting! I've never been skinny and don't ever expect to be, so I had resigned myself to being overweight. But I felt an urge to go to your meeting on health and weight management, and I'm glad I did. I've lost fifteen pounds as of this morning, and I'm not looking back!

I've been telling all my friends and co-workers about your idea for losing weight. I've changed my snacking habits and have started enjoying almonds. I'm grazing during the day at work on healthy foods instead of the chocolates and other candies hanging around the office. I am currently only one pound behind my target weight for this week.

The only bad news is that I've lost the same two pounds *five* times!

I love the freedom the Jerusalem Diet gives me to eat what I want on good days, and I'm getting better about eating fruits, veggies, nuts, and seeds on the "oops" days. Thank you for having the courage to bring a sensitive topic out in the open for us. Thank you for giving us an enjoyable diet. I didn't know there was such a thing!

Sincerely,

Ginger

us have a hormone called leptin, which helps control our appetite. Leptin is produced by fat cells, and it helps the brain know whether the body is full or needs food. Keeping leptin levels consistent is crucial to countering weight gain.

What does this have to do with sleep? Well, the body's production of hormones is affected by sleep. Normally, leptin levels rise when we sleep, so the body feels sated during the night hours. The reason you don't often wake up in the middle of the night needing a snack is that your body's leptin is telling the brain there is plenty of food in storage. If you deprive your body of sleep, you may develop a shortage of leptin. And if you aren't producing enough leptin, your body may start asking for food it doesn't really need.[1]

This information contains an important lesson for those of us who have to watch our weight: to really take care of our bodies, we must make sure we get proper rest.

Because of leptin production, eating and sleeping have another important connection as well: if we eat early in the evening rather than near bedtime, we'll sleep better and help our bodies maintain reasonable hunger levels. Dr. John de Castro, a researcher at the University of Texas at El Paso who devotes much of his study to our eating habits, has suggested there is a real link between eating early and losing weight. Late at night our body expects to be sleeping, and our body's satiation mechanism may not function as well as it does earlier in the day. If we snack or eat meals late in the evening, we may be prone to eat too much because our body is less likely to signal that it is full.[2]

So eat early in the evening. When I do that regularly, I sleep better. I wake up hungry, and when I wake up hungry, I eat a better breakfast.

What if you are so hungry that you can't sleep? A bedtime snack can do the trick, especially if you're strategic about it. Eat something with tryptophan in it—the amino acid that helps your brain produce serotonin, which is a relaxing agent. Drink warm milk, eat a couple of slices of turkey, or—in good

Jerusalem Diet fashion—nibble on peanuts. They all contain tryptophan. Cottage cheese, yogurt, ice cream, chicken, soy beans, and tuna have tryptophan too.

But as much as possible, eat early and sleep well. Your body will thank you.

CHAPTER 18

Q and A on the Jerusalem Diet

I did the best I could, but there are some topics not covered well or at all in this book. Here are questions I've received. I hope my answers will clarify matters.

Q: *What if your Fat Day doesn't work? What if you go through a day of fruits, vegetables, nuts, seeds, water, and an hour of exercise and still don't hit your target the next day?*

A: For a typical person, in order for this to happen, you would have to eat a wheelbarrow full of real food! So take another day, and don't gorge yourself on fruits, vegetables, nuts, and seeds. Drink enough water to pee pale, and increase the intensity of your exercise. You'll do great. If, though, you can't get to your target weight, you might have a medical condition that needs to be checked by a physician. But for the vast majority of people, one day will work, and two days will work for sure. (Uh, unless you cheat.) Remember, rocky road ice cream, even though it has nuts, doesn't qualify for a Fat Day snack.

Q: *How do Fat Days work with family dinners when one person is having a Fat Day and another is not?*

A: The person on the Fat Day should stick to fruits, vegetables, nuts, seeds, and water. It's not hard. Have a salad with water. Let others eat normally. Remember, the Jerusalem Diet requires a day of discipline.

Q: *Do you think the Jerusalem Diet is safe for children?*

A: Are you kidding? Every nutritional program I've seen for kids says they need to eat more fruits and vegetables. Childhood obesity is increasingly a problem because of bad food and drinks and the lack of exercise. My guess is that the Jerusalem Diet would be great for normal kids dealing with weight and diet problems. If you have special concerns, though, talk with a pediatrician. After hearing about the Jerusalem Diet, most doctors like it so much that they go on it themselves, because they are like me: busy and not able to spend hours in the gym. Many doctors have put their patients on the Jerusalem Diet. I don't know of any pediatricians doing that, but I suspect that pediatricians would be happy to have their overweight patients use a simple system that includes exercise and eating more fruits and vegetables, nuts and seeds while laying off junk food and sodas for a few days.

Q: *You say your family history suggests a propensity toward obesity, but you have not had a lifelong weight problem. What about those of us who have? My body does not recover from binges in the same way yours does. If I splurge on sweets, I may have to have five Fat Days in a row to get back on target. Help!*

A: Fat Days are not bad. They are not punishment. They are good for you. You may need to adjust your weight-loss portion of the plan to lose one pound every two weeks instead of each week. Actually, a doctor friend of mine thinks one pound a week is too fast for some people, and I agree. So slow down. If you've been overweight all your life, then your frame, your skin, your body will need time to adjust as you lose weight.

I did not overemphasize intensity of exercise in this book, because I want to encourage obese people to include exercise in their lifestyle. Some physical activity is better than none. But for most people, a little more punch in their exercise will help. Remember to include both cardiovascular and resistance exercise. The cardio will help your circulatory system, which is vital. The resistance exercises will build muscle, which is key to sustained weight control. Drink enough water to pee pale, and don't cheat for twenty-four hours. I don't know of anyone, anytime, anywhere who ever needed five Fat Days to get under control. Nope, I don't believe it.

Q: *You say that if you mess up and enjoy some decadent food, even on a Fat Day, you forgive yourself and pick up again later. Easy for you to say! What if I have a hard time forgiving myself? How do you learn to do that?*

A: No doubt about it, guilt can play a positive role. But maybe in your case you need to be more careful on Fat Days. Don't mess up. I'm a strong believer in forgiveness, so I don't have any problem repenting and getting back on track. If you can't, though, then don't get off track to begin with.

Q: *Should I write each day's target weight and actual weight on the calendar? How should I keep track of progress?*

A: When you are on your weight-loss schedule, you'll have the same target weight all week. Be sure to write the number on your calendar so you'll know that is the target weight for the week. However, if it helps you to put your target weight on every day for seven days—go for it. Then you will have a daily reminder that your goal is to reduce that number by one pound before the seven days are up. You need not, though, write your actual weight every day unless you want to. When you weigh yourself first thing in the morning, you know if you are okay that day or if you are having a Fat Day. That's all you need to know. If you are okay, enjoy the day, but try not to eat so much that you'll have a Fat Day tomorrow. If you are having a Fat Day, then enjoy the day by strengthening your body with good food (fruits, vegetables, nuts, and seeds), proper hydration (drink plenty of water), and appropriate exercise (at least an hour).

Q: *What if—in typical dieter's fashion—I lose weight the first few weeks of the Jerusalem Diet but then plateau and fail to progress toward my ideal weight? What's up with that?*

A: Start again tomorrow morning. It's true; if you don't do it, it won't work. You need to be intentional. This doesn't work if you don't do it. However, if you are plateauing, you might have discovered your natural weight.

Keep trying and don't cheat. If there is no movement in your weight, and you are over your ideal weight, talk with your doctor to see if something else is affecting your weight.

Q: *You say to weigh yourself at the same time every day, but most of your examples are first thing in the morning. Does it matter when you weigh yourself? You also say that our weight fluctuates more than we might think—so how does this figure into the daily weigh-in?*

A: As you go through the day, you gain weight, which is why weighing at the same time each day provides a consistent plumb line for your progress. I like to weigh myself first thing in the morning either right after I go to the bathroom or after I shower and dry off—just before I get dressed. Weighing myself at this point in the day is what determines if I'm having a Fat Day. In addition, sometimes I'll weigh myself in the late afternoon to see if I can splurge on dinner or a late snack. I typically lose one to two pounds while I sleep. So if I'm at my ideal (or target) weight at 6:00 p.m., I know I have some wiggle room. If I'm two pounds over my ideal (or target) weight, I need to be careful, or I'll have a Fat Day tomorrow.

Q: *When weighing myself, how should I deal with weight fluctuations due to water retention? In other words, how do I think about my daily weight as it fluctuates due to menstruation, eating salty foods, vigorous exercise, or other factors? This is particularly of interest to women, whose weight fluctuates much more than men's.*

A: When a woman goes through her monthly cycle and has a heavy day because of water retention, it is actually a good time for her—healthwise—to have a day of real food, water, and exercise. She'll feel better, and many women who stay with the plan regardless of where they are in their monthly cycle don't experience so many issues with PMS. Salt does help your body retain water, which is often good. If it's excessive and affects your weight, you should have a day of good food, additional water to cleanse your system, and some exercise. If, because of exercise, you are dehydrated, that will balance out in a day. I drink a glass of water before I go to bed so my body can enjoy the water as I sleep. (I know—a weird thought!)

The Jerusalem Diet is specifically designed so you won't inadvertently lose weight by becoming dehydrated. That would be horrible for you. Instead, do the opposite. Let the water help your system work well so you lose the excess weight and are healthy. Your body needs the water. Drink good, clean, fresh water.

Q: *What is the significance of body mass index (BMI)? Why does the Jerusalem Diet focus solely on weight and not on BMI or body-fat percentage?*

A: In fact, the scale I weigh myself on attempts to give a body-fat percentage in addition to weight. I think BMI is important, but in most people it automatically adjusts as they drop excess weight and build muscle through exercise. In Covert Bailey's excellent book *The Ultimate Fit or Fat*, he gives the easiest methods of determining BMI with specific goals for fitness. I think, though, if you'll lose a pound every week or two until you reach your ideal weight, and exercise in order to build additional muscle, you'll find your BMI moving in the right direction.

Q: *One theory says, "Don't weigh yourself. Focus on waistline inches." What do you make of this?*

A: The objective of this idea is to keep people from losing fat without also toning up and building muscle. I agree, which is why on a Fat Day we have the hour of exercise. I don't like the "don't weigh yourself" suggestion, though. It doesn't work for people like me. I need a daily reminder of where I am, and when I put on my clothes, that provides me with incentive about my waistline. I love it when my clothes are comfortable. I hate it when they are too snug. So, in fact, if we monitor our weight every day and put on clothes every day, we get the best of both worlds.

Q: *Is it okay to eat red meat? Enjoy in moderation?*

A: Yes, enjoy in moderation. Red meat is an excellent source of protein and many other nutrients your body needs. Shop for good meat. Do your research. It will benefit you. I'm concerned about some of the modern cattle feeding methods, so be informed about the meat you eat. Consult your doctor if you have any questions regarding specific health issues and red meat.

Q: *What do you think about the decision many people make to be vegetarians?*

A: I'm fine with it as long as they supplement their diets so they are eating what their bodies need. Some are vegetarians because they love animals and don't want to eat meat. Others do it for health reasons. I'm relaxed on the topic, but I think we're best if we eat a large variety of foods so our bodies can get what they need and we can enjoy life more. Relax! Eat! And, as we do, if we eat better food, our bodies will be healthier.

Q: *How important is label reading? Some products that are marketed as being healthy may not be as good for you as they say. Certain sweetened dried fruits, salted seeds and nuts, granola bars, trail mixes, and fruit and vegetable smoothies come to mind.*

A: No doubt about it, knowing what we put into our bodies is the point. It's a good idea to avoid refined sugar and trans fats (at least according to the latest nutritional information). Some processed foods contain excess salt and flavor enhancers that are difficult for our bodies to process/digest. Remember, generally speaking, if we eat food in its natural state, we are better off.

Q: *Do you recommend eating five to six smaller meals each day or three squares?*

A: Grazing is better than three solid meals a day, but it's hard for most people to eat this way. If you are like this, make your meals smaller and snack on good foods between meals.

Q: *I hate to be pessimistic, but what do I do about nutrition and exercise during times of intense stress? What if a family member dies or has a prolonged illness? What if I'm in a particularly busy period of life?*

A: In my experience, exercise is one of the best things you can do in the midst of stress. I love to jog because it releases tension, gives me an opportunity to think, and strengthens my body. It's excellent. If you are in a particularly busy period of life, then the Jerusalem Diet will work for you. The main thing is to watch your food intake by eating smaller portions and better food.

Q: *You say to lose no more than one pound per week because our bodies have a hard time adjusting to quick changes. But I've dieted before and tended to slim down pretty quickly. What if I lose five to ten pounds in the first couple of weeks?*

A: You will pay. Your body will punish you. And if it worked so well, why are you reading this? I think I might know. You didn't keep the extra weight off. In the Jerusalem Diet plan, you can do a crash diet if you like, and you can, in fact, lose significant weight quickly. But create your overall Jerusalem Diet plan so that you'll keep the weight off. Some do use crash plans to lose and the Jerusalem Diet to maintain. That's fine with me, but I cringe at the thought of transitioning your body chemistry and function too quickly. No doubt it can be done. But slow, steady transitions will service you better. Hopefully, what you're really after is a healthy lifestyle change that results in your ideal body weight and fitness.

Q: *You don't make a huge deal out of salted versus unsalted varieties of nuts and seeds. Can you say more about this?*

A: Most people can eat what they prefer. Salt is good for us. Excessive amounts of salt aren't. But for normal people, if they eat salted nuts on their Fat Days, they are also drinking water. If they are adequately hydrated, they will be fine. No worries. Relax. Eat. Enjoy. If your doctor has instructed you to limit your salt intake, do it. But most people don't have this concern.

Q: *On Fat Days, is it okay to have a veggie sandwich with bread?*

A: You can, but the bread isn't going to help you. I'd ditch the bread and eat the rest.

Q: *You're a pastor, so tell me—if the Bible is supposed to be a book for all ages, why does it say so little about nutrition, health, and exercise? These issues significantly affect well-being and quality of life in the modern age, so why doesn't the Bible offer more direction?*

A: The Bible gives us everything we need to know about spiritual life and many principles about morality, relationships, and practical living. It was written, though, in a time when people walked all day, every day, while eating unprocessed food. Only the hyper-wealthy were fat, so being fat was a status symbol. The vast majority of people in Bible times exercised more than our most avid exercise fanatics today. As a result, lack of exercise wasn't an issue then. In addition, if you have traveled to the Middle East, you know the diet there is much more natural than ours is in the West. People living in the Middle East naturally consume fruits, vegetables, nuts, and seeds. They enjoy yogurt, water, and exercise. So I think I would take a little different spin on this than your question implies. Maybe the Jerusalem Diet is appropriately named. The food and exercise from Bible times may be exactly what it moves people toward.

Q: *Do the dietary restrictions in both the Old and New Testaments play any part in the Jerusalem Diet? For instance, what about pork?*

A: I think the biblical mandates are good. Scientists are finding that biblical exhortations on this and other subjects are not just random but are there for a reason. Heed the Good Book. But on the Jerusalem Diet, on a Fat Day stick to fruits, vegetables, nuts, seeds, water, and exercise. In doing this, you'll not violate any biblical mandates. Then, on your okay days, if you want to avoid pork and other "forbidden foods," it will serve you well.

Q: *I am a recovering bulimic. I have not had a bulimic episode for two years, but I'm not sure about dieting. While using other diets in the past, I would become frustrated at my lack of progress and start purging. What is the Jerusalem Diet way of dealing with this?*

A: It's slow, it's easy, and it's effective. It doesn't make you think about your diet and food all the time. It allows you to live without being consumed with your body or your looks. You'll neither go hungry nor feel condemned for eating what you like to eat. It's the diet that makes people happy. I think you'll like it.

Q: *Give it to me straight—how strict are your fruits, vegetables, nuts, and seeds days? No yogurt dips for fruit? No salad dressing?*

A: As I said earlier, on a Fat Day I often have yogurt just before I go to bed. And, oops, I always have salad dressing. Good question. You caught me!

Q: *Okay, no biggie. But what kind of salad dressing? Seriously. Not just any kind is okay, right?*

A: I eat the kind I like. This system works so well, I doubt that the salad dressing will throw you off. Back off the volume of food and enjoy the flavor.

Q: *On non–Fat Days, what about potatoes or white bread?*

A: You can eat them, but if you eat too much, you increase your likelihood of having a Fat Day the next day. If you're fit, you can eat more. If you're fat, it will make you worse. But you don't have to eliminate them. I like potatoes and bread. On the bread note, ditch white bread 100 percent. Retrain yourself to buy whole-grain bread. I only eat white bread when I am at Burger King or some place like that. At home it's whole-grain bread.

Q: *At one point you mentioned making a big sandwich for lunch, but at another point you noted the potential problem with deli meats and said you preferred salads for lunch. I've long wondered about the deli meat issue. What do you really think about deli meats? What about sandwiches versus salads for lunch?*

A: I love it all. I love lots of things that are potential problems, such as shrimp. Don't let potential problems discourage you, just ease in the direction of eating better foods more often and problem foods less often. It's the trajectory of your life that matters. Your body is pretty incredible. It will handle a variety of foods just fine as long as once in a while you give it real food, refreshing water, and exercise.

Q: *When you start eating like this, does your body go through a kind of cleansing? I ask because after my first couple of days on the Jerusalem Diet, I felt like I was coming down with the flu!*

A: If your body is used to being fed junk all the time, it will readjust with real food. If you are addicted to caffeine or sugar, you may get a headache or leg ache. Take a pain reliever, but stick with the plan. (I'll never forget the first time I had blueberries for breakfast. They are great in every way, unless your body isn't used to them.) You might have mild stomach or intestinal problems, but take the plunge anyway. Note, though, that on the Jerusalem Diet, you only eat fruits, vegetables, nuts, and seeds, and drink water, and exercise on Fat Days. You shouldn't have two consecutive days of this unless you cheat or you consider rolling over in bed an exercise.

Q: *I've been a runner for years, but recently I've been encouraged to take up walking because jogging is hard on the knees. Do you have a view on this? I would hate to stop running.*

A: Get good shoes, make sure you are adequately hydrated, run on soft surfaces, and when you run inside, use a high-quality treadmill or one of the new machines that are low impact. But it's true; your joints would prefer a brisk walk. Again, moderation is a good idea.

Q: *What is the significance of having active hobbies, such as biking or gardening, instead of sedentary hobbies, such as crafts or watching television?*

A: Movement. If you don't move, you will die. Besides that, active hobbies are good for your mind because you have time to think while doing them, whereas your brain is less active when you're watching television than it is when you're sleeping.

Q: *What is the reason for waiting until I've reached two-thirds of my weight-loss goal before beginning daily push-ups, sit-ups, and squats?*

A: It's because most people need to lose weight before they can do these exercises effectively. If you start at your two-thirds point, you'll be very pleased. If you start at the beginning, the odds of getting discouraged and quitting are very high, because this is a marathon. If you'll use the system, the chances of your loving your life for the rest of your life go sky high. If you try to go to college after finishing the first grade, you might get discouraged. One step at a time, and you'll love the Jerusalem Diet.

Q: *Why do you say that I should wait until I reach my ideal weight to begin resistance training? And since muscle weighs more than fat, will my ideal weight need to adjust as I gain muscle?*

A: You don't have to wait. You might want to start resistance training at the two-thirds point, along with the daily exercise, to keep yourself toned. Muscle burns calories; fat doesn't. Therefore, movement stimulates metabolism; rest doesn't. Muscle does weigh more than fat, which is why, when you reach your ideal weight and begin resistance training, you'll still lose fat in order to compensate for the weight of the muscle you're gaining. So, on the Jerusalem Diet, you lose fat during your weight-loss phase. At two-thirds of the way to your goal, start push-ups, sit-ups (or crunches), and squats (never lower than a 90-degree angle with your knees). Then, once you reach your ideal weight, start resistance training in earnest, and you'll continue to lose fat and gain muscle. If you are measuring your body mass index, you'll notice fitness increasing significantly at this stage. Also at this stage you will love the way your body shape continues to improve. This is a great plan.

Q: *Are you really that obsessed with junk food and Mountain Dew? Early in the book it sounds like you are addicted to the stuff, but later it sounds like you are a pretty healthy eater most of the time. Which is it?*

A: Both are true. It depends upon when you catch me.

Q: *If people have diabetes or blood-sugar issues, should they eliminate fruit on Fat Days?*

A: Most don't need to, but if they are concerned, they should ask their doctor.

Q: *Tea is a superfood. What if you add sweetener to it? Does that make it less than super?*

A: Use raw sugar or honey, and you'll be fine.

Q: *I heard that soy is no longer all that super of a food. What do you make of some research that says soy can lead to Alzheimer's?*

A: There is an ongoing debate about this, so go easy on soy. Personally, I can't stand soy! But if you can, go easy on the tofu and other soy products. Don't overdo it on health-food fads. Just eat more good food than bad food, and as time passes, eat more and more real food. Drink water, exercise, and let your body serve you. If you take care of it, it will have greater potential to take care of you.

CHAPTER 19

Be Nice!

Imagine this: you've been on the Jerusalem Diet for a few weeks—maybe more than a month. So far so good. You've slipped up here and there, not having time to exercise as much as you'd like and having visions of Double Stuf Oreos appear in your dreams like never before. But you've lost four pounds. You feel invigorated. You are getting the hang of this. Nuts and seeds have replaced Tootsie Rolls for midafternoon snacks. Morning fruit and vegetable juices have replaced four-shot lattes. For the most part.

But one night you binge on fried chicken and banana cream pie, relishing every bite. You know you might be over your target weight the next day, but it's worth it for a couple of hours of kicking back with comfort food and a great old black-and-white movie.

The next morning you are indeed over your target. No big deal—you'll just enjoy a grapefruit breakfast, a salad lunch, almonds for snacking, and another salad for dinner.

But during the day some friends call and invite you over for dinner. Tonight's the only night that will work for everyone. You accept. When you get there, you find lamb curry with basmati rice for the main course, followed by homemade vanilla ice cream with fresh berries for dessert.

What do you do? You could say, "No, thanks! I'll just pick at the salad. I'm a pound over today, you know."

Or you could smile, be thankful, and eat what is served.

You know what I think you should do.

Don't be a Jerusalem Diet prude. Don't be a South Beach snob. Don't be annoying about Atkins. Be nice. Eat what is served, and when you walk out the door, you can go back on your plan. Don't gorge yourself. Eat a reasonable portion of what is served, and you might be pleasantly surprised the next morning. The scale news may not be as bad as feared. You still have your life on a new and good trajectory. There are millions of nondieters out there, and that's okay. You used to be one of them too.

There have been many times when I've been in people's homes on a Fat Day and have been disappointed to be served cheeseburgers or pork loin. There have been business lunches where the man I was meeting said, "We've just got to go to this restaurant for ribs!" and I've had to swallow my healthy intentions and just deal with it in order to be polite (as if I minded all that much).

Here's what I do in those situations: I don't overeat. Because I saw the number on the scale that morning, I'm more conscious of the fact that it's a Fat Day. I chew more slowly and eat less. I stick with water if possible. And not once—never—has a situation like that kept me from getting back on target the next day.

When situations like this happen, I remember a tip I got from my friend Terry Felber. He taught me years ago that it's better to eat calories than to drink them. So when I'm close to the edge, I would rather eat food that isn't exactly on the plan and drink water than drink a Mountain Dew loaded with calories and be over the next morning.

I hope that the Jerusalem Diet causes the sun to shine on you. I hope it liberates you to appreciate food and enjoy your life more than before. But I also hope it helps you liberate others—not by preaching the gospel of weight loss all the time but by showing them how to have an appropriate relationship with food and health.

Have you noticed the overall tone of the testimonies you've read throughout this book? I love how soft-spoken many of them are. They are thrilled about how much better they're doing, but they're a little tentative, because food has always been hard for them to talk about. It's as though they think talking about their success too eagerly will cause it to go away.

Diet is a touchy issue. People often feel bad about the way they look. They carry guilt about how they're not exercising enough or how they can't seem to drive past a Papa John's without craving cheese bread. If they're obviously overweight, it's no secret to them; you certainly don't need to point it out. Even if they just *feel* overweight when they aren't, that, too, can be burdensome.

So I say go easy on people. Be loving. Be sensitive. If you want to share your diet tips with others, do it in a way that can be received. If you talk about your new eating and exercising habits in a way that makes friends flinch, take note and try talking about it differently. Some people may be eager to hear your advice; others may not be in a position to receive what you have to say.

At times you may need to keep your advice to yourself. If you've just read this book or *The Maker's Diet* or Dr. Atkins or some educational nutrition guide, you may be so pumped full of knowledge that you feel you're about to burst. But if you come home and see your spouse munching on a Fig Newton, don't say, "Oh, let me tell you about what that's doing in your body!" Don't watch your wife or husband go to the fridge for a soda and offer, "Why don't you try a bottled water instead?"

I like the Jerusalem Diet because it's a slow, steady change in the trajectory of our lives. If people say, "Are you losing weight?" the appropriate response is, "I'm trying to maintain my health. I found a plan that you might like." If they ask how you're trying to improve your health, explain the concepts of the Jerusalem Diet. Tell them, "My goal is to achieve my ideal weight, improve my potential for health, look and feel as good as I can, and live a great life."

I don't want to be overweight.

I don't want to be unnecessarily sick.

I want to be as alive as I can.

When I tell people about the Jerusalem Diet, they often laugh and say, "Is that possible?" or, "Are you serious?"

I always respond, "I know. It's ridiculous. But I need a plan that keeps me in line without having to be disciplined for more than twenty-four hours at a time. I need to be able to eat egg rolls and drink a Coke or Pepsi from time to time." People like the life-giving, lighthearted attitude of the diet. It's not threatening. It's doable. And after they hear about it a time or two, it begins to make sense.

You'll remember the nutritionist who told my friend that this plan wouldn't work. My take? I think the nutritionist needs this plan. He needs to be liberated from rigid diets. He espouses the expert opinion, but he doesn't know what people are actually willing and able to do.

Something is better than *nothing.* More is better than less. Some exercise is better than no exercise. Regular exercise is better than sporadic exercise. Some real food is better than no real food. Some water with some coffee is better than all coffee and no water.

We live on a continuum. Most of our lives we are somewhere between perfect health and disease and immobility. We're somewhere between a bale of hay and refined flour. We want to move toward health but not miss out on the wonderful pleasures of life. That's okay. We're somewhere in between, gradually working toward a better place.

And most of us have friends and family members for whom we are concerned. There are people whom we want to contribute to—people who need advice on health and fitness. But we need to love them and care for them in a way they can receive. We need to be gentle and offer hope, not add to their burdens and fears.

I'm so excited about this book that when I travel, I carry copies to give away. I see people all the time who are too fat and, because of their schedules, don't believe they can reduce their weight and become more fit. This plan is the solution.

So lighten up! Do what you can. Help others without making them feel as if they have to have a perfect body and eat perfect food in order to be acceptable. Love life, love your friends, love your body. Cooperate with the realities of life, but at the same time, nudge your own life and the lives of your friends in a positive direction. Be nice. Don't be a snob, and life will get better and better for you.

❦

So that's it—the Jerusalem Diet.

Now you have a plan that works for busy people. It's easy, doable, and best of all, it really works. It a simple plan that can benefit just about everyone. It's healthy, it will reset the trajectory of your life, and it will walk you slowly through reshaping your body, adjusting your weight to its ideal, lowering your body fat to a reasonable level, and jump-starting your metabolism. The Jerusalem Diet gives room for steady progress as you read other diet, exercise, and nutrition books and articles. This is a total life plan that will give you greater hope for a happier future. You will never need a crash exercise or diet program again. Weigh yourself every morning, and live that day according to the plan.

Now let's go to Dairy Queen!

Resources

Reading Resources

Agatston, Arthur. T*he South Beach Diet: The Delicious, Doctor-Designed, Foolproof Plan for Fast and Healthy Weight Loss.* Emmaus, PA: Rodale, 2003.

Atkins, Robert C. *Dr. Atkins Diet Revolution: The High Calorie Way to Stay Thin Forever.* New York: D. McKay, 1972.

Bailey, Covert. *The Ultimate Fit or Fat: Get in Shape and Stay in Shape with America's Best-Loved and Most Effective Fitness Teacher.* Boston: Houghton Mifflin, 1999.

Bailey, Covert, and Ronda Gates. *Smart Eating: Choosing Wisely, Living Lean.* Boston: Houghton Mifflin, 1996.

Cooper, Kenneth H. *The Aerobics Program for Total Well-Being: Exercise, Diet, and Emotional Balance.* New York: M. Evans, 1982.

Cooper, Kenneth H. *Controlling Cholesterol: Dr. Kenneth H. Cooper's Preventive Medicine Program.* New York: Bantam Books, 1988.

Cooper, Kenneth H. *Faith-Based Fitness: The Medical Program That Uses Spiritual Motivation to Achieve Maximum Health and Add Years to Your Life.* Nashville: Thomas Nelson, 1995.

Cooper, Kenneth H. *Regaining the Power of Youth at Any Age: Startling New Evidence from the Doctor Who Brought Us Aerobics, Controlling Cholesterol and the Antioxidant Revolution.* Nashville: Thomas Nelson, 1998.

D'Adamo, Peter J., with Catherine Whitney. *Eat Right 4 Your Type: The Individualized Diet Solution to Staying Healthy, Living Longer & Achieving Your Ideal Weight.* New York: G. P. Putnam's Sons, 1996.

Herbert, Victor, and Genell J. Subak-Sharpe, eds. *Total Nutrition: The Only Guide You'll Ever Need.* New York: St. Martin's, 1995.

Pratt, Steven G., and Kathy Matthews. *SuperFoods Rx: Fourteen Foods That Will Change Your Life.* New York: William Morrow, 2004.

Rubin, Jordan S. *The Maker's Diet.* Lake Mary, FL: Siloam, 2004.

Russell, Rex. *What the Bible Says About Healthy Living: Three Biblical Principles That Will Change Your Diet and Improve Your Health.* Ventura, CA: Regal, 1996.

Willett, Walter C., with P. J. Skerrett. *Eat, Drink, and Be Healthy: The Harvard Medical School Guide to Healthy Eating.* New York: Free Press, 2005.

Blenders and Juicers

Jack LaLanne Power Juicer—http://www.asseenontvnetwork.com/vcc/tristar/powerjuicer/132971/

Vita-Mix—www.vitamix.com

Online Ideal-Weight Calculators

http://www.active.com/calculators/idealweight_calc_togo.cfm

http://www.fitnessonline.com/tools/idealweight/

http://www.halls.md/ideal-weight/body.htm

http://www.healthstatus.com/calculate/iwc

Notes

Chapter 4: All Diets Work (but None Work for Me)

1. Steven G. Pratt and Kathy Matthews, *SuperFoods Rx: Fourteen Foods That Will Change Your Life* (New York: William Morrow, 2004).

2. Robert C. Atkins, "The Great Nutrition Debate," Millennium Lecture Series, U.S. Department of Agriculture, Washington DC, February 24, 2000.

Chapter 5: Change Your Life…Slowly

1. Centers for Disease Control and Prevention, Genomics and Disease Prevention, "Obesity and Genetics: What We Know, What We Don't Know and What It Means," www.cdc.gov/genomics/info/perspectives/files/obesknow.htm.

2. Walter C. Willett with P. J. Skerrett, *Eat, Drink, and Be Healthy: The Harvard Medical School Guide to Healthy Eating* (New York: Free Press, 2001), 43.

3. Victor Herbert and Genell J. Subak-Sharpe, eds., *Total Nutrition: The Only Guide You'll Ever Need* (New York: St. Martin's, 1995), 220.

4. Phillip Rhodes, "Belly-Off All-Stars," *Men's Health,* June 20, 2005, www.menshealth.com/cda/article.do?site=MensHealth&channel=weight.loss&category=belly.off.club&conitem=5953f8548b594010VgnVCM200000cee793cd____&page=0&pageLocation=true.

5. Rex Russell, *What the Bible Says About Healthy Living: Three Biblical Principles That Will Change Your Diet and Improve Your Health* (Ventura, CA: Regal, 1996).

6. Lifespan, "The National Weight Control Registry Research Findings," 2001, www.nwcr.ws/Research/01.htm.

Chapter 6: Change Your Home's Culture

1. Walter Willett, interview, "The Diet Wars," *Frontline,* Public Broadcasting System, January 9, 2004.

2. Willett, interview, "The Diet Wars."

Chapter 7: Change Your Life's Trajectory

1. Eileen H. Shinn and Carlos Poston, "Why We Are Overweight: Genes vs. Lifestyle," *Detroit News,* 2005, http://detroitnews.healthology.com/focus_article.asp?f=beyond_dieting&c=envsgenes.

2. "Legislation Proposed to Increase Americans' Consumption of Fruits and Vegetables," *Food and Drink Weekly* 9, no. 25 (June 30, 2003): 1.

Chapter 8: A Day on the Jerusalem Diet

1. Jennifer Warner, "Yogurt May Help Burn Fat, Promote Weight Loss," *WebMDHealth,* March 17, 2005, http://my.webmd.com/content/article/102/106625.htm.

Chapter 9: Weigh Yourself Daily

1. Walter C. Willett with P. J. Skerrett, *Eat, Drink, and Be Healthy: The Harvard Medical School Guide to Healthy Eating* (New York: Free Press, 2001), 35.

Chapter 10: Eat Fat-Day Foods

1. Victor Herbert and Genell J. Subak-Sharpe, eds., *Total Nutrition: The Only Guide You'll Ever Need* (New York: St. Martin's, 1995), 19.

2. Damian McNamara, "African Americans Might Benefit from DASH Approach," *Family Practice News* 33, no. 13 (July 1, 2003): 9.

3. Herbert and Subak-Sharpe, *Total Nutrition,* 60–61.

4. Herbert and Subak-Sharpe, *Total Nutrition,* 686–87.

5. Herbert and Subak-Sharpe, *Total Nutrition,* 686.

6. Walter C. Willett with P. J. Skerrett, *Eat, Drink, and Be Healthy: The Harvard Medical School Guide to Healthy Eating* (New York: Free Press, 2001), 114–15.

7. Willett with Skerrett, *Eat, Drink, and Be Healthy,* 119.

8. Herbert and Subak-Sharpe, *Total Nutrition,* 700.

9. Herbert and Subak-Sharpe, *Total Nutrition,* 684.

10. Herbert and Subak-Sharpe, *Total Nutrition,* 684.

11. Richard N. Fogoros, "Say Nuts to Heart Disease," About.com, May 4, 2001, http://heartdisease.about.com/cs/riskfactors/a/nuts.htm.

12. Joan Sabate et al., "Effects of Walnuts on Serum Lipid Levels and Blood Pressure in Normal Men," *New England Journal of Medicine* 328, no. 9 (March 4, 1993): 603–7.

13. Steven G. Pratt and Kathy Matthews, *SuperFoods Rx: Fourteen Foods That Will Change Your Life* (New York: William Morrow, 2004), 182.

Chapter 13: Break Addictions

1. Walter C. Willett with P. J. Skerrett, *Eat, Drink, and Be Healthy: The Harvard Medical School Guide to Healthy Eating* (New York: Free Press, 2001), 132–33.

2. "Caffeine Withdrawal Recognized as a Disorder," *Johns Hopkins Medicine,* September 29, 2004, www.hopkinsmedicine.org/Press_releases/2004/09_29_04.html.

Chapter 16: Drink Your Fruits and Vegetables

1. Walter C. Willett with P. J. Skerrett, *Eat, Drink, and Be Healthy: The Harvard Medical School Guide to Healthy Eating* (New York: Free Press, 2001), 129–31.

2. Willett with Skerrett, *Eat, Drink, and Be Healthy,* 128.

Chapter 17: Eat Early and Get a Good Night's Rest

1. "Too Little Sleep Combined with Holiday Overeating May Increase Risk of Obesity," National Sleep Foundation, November 18, 2004, http://sleepfoundation.org/press/index.php?secid=&id=82.

2. John M. de Castro, "The Time of Day of Food Intake Influences Overall Intake in Humans," Human Nutrition and Metabolism, American Society for Nutritional Sciences, Nutrition.org, January 2004, www.nutrition.org/cgi/content/abstract/134/1/104?maxtoshow= &HITS=10&hits=10&RESULTFORMAT=&author1=de+Castro&full text=eating%2C+overeating%2C+diet&searchid=1080847892318_ 5545&stored_search=&FIRSTINDEX=0&sortspec=relevance& journalcode=nutrition.

Index

About the Author

Ted Haggard is president of the thirty-million-member National Association of Evangelicals (NAE), the largest evangelical group in America. He is also founder and senior pastor of the eleven-thousand-member New Life Church in Colorado Springs, Colorado.

Ted founded and serves as the president of both the Association of Life-Giving Churches, a network of local churches, and worldprayerteam.org, the only real-time global prayer network. He is also the author of seven books, including the best-selling *Primary Purpose*.

Ted and his wife, Gayle, live in Colorado Springs with their five children.

For more information, visit the following Web sites:

• New Life Church: www.newlifechurch.org

• The National Association of Evangelicals: www.nae.net

• The Association of Life-Giving Churches: www.lifegivingchurch.org

• World Prayer Team: www.worldprayerteam.org

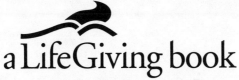
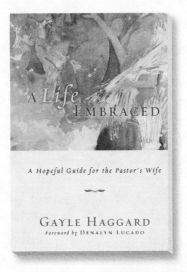
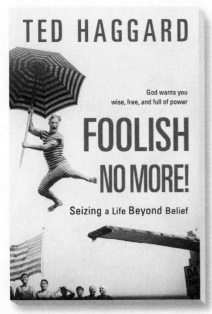
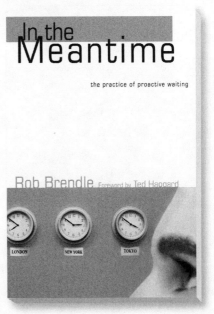
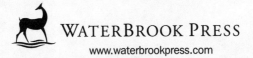